Get Help

Get Help

A guide for social workers to the management of illness in the community

Primrose Halliburton
and Kate Quelch

Tavistock Publications
London and New York

First published in 1981 by
Tavistock Publications Ltd
11 New Fetter Lane, London EC4P 4EE

Printed in the United States of America

British Library Cataloguing in Publication Data

Halliburton, Primrose
Get help: a guide for social workers to the management of illness in the community. – (Social science paperbacks)
1. Care of the sick 2. Social service
I. Title II. Quelch, Kate
362.1'4'024362 HV687

ISBN 0-422-77560-6
ISBN 0-422-77570-3 Pbk

Contents

We thank
Our advisers, Miss K. M. Lee and Dr W. B. Wright, for their knowledge and encouragement
Our colleagues for their help and generosity
Our secretary for her efficiency and forbearance.

Preface

Since the upheavals of local government and health service re-organization in 1974, and the considerable debate that surrounded the place of and responsibility for social work in the new health service, the two authors of this book have moved from their former hospital bases to work within the wider context of a social service department with its involvement in residential and domiciliary care, as well as field social work.

They brought with them a wealth of expertise and experience and since then have acquired considerable knowledge and understanding of the problems and needs of their colleagues throughout the social work profession. The result is this book, which will make a real and valuable contribution to the resources available to both generic social workers and those specialist social workers who, from time to time, become involved in less familiar fields.

JOHN LLEWELLYN
Director of Social Services,
Oxfordshire County Council.

Foreword

Each profession has its own culture and language and each trains its own students in cloistered isolation. Students emerge from their training able to understand their own language, but unable to communicate with members of other professions. They may recognize, in the abstract, words used by others and may even become familiar with some of their terminology. Few, however, work for a sufficient amount of time, or sufficiently close to other professional groups to really learn their language.

To expect that things might be otherwise, that a common professional language might develop, seems now, in the manner of the Esperantists, to be hopelessly Utopian. In fact just as there is an increasing need for discrete cultural groups to retain their own language, so distinct professional groups are developing and perpetuating their own particular modes of expression, often in a way inaccessible to others.

This monolingualism amongst professionals in the health and social services is highly regrettable. The authors of this book have learned the language of the health service professionals, and their experience is distilled for those who are new to their work as social workers, or who may never have the opportunity of long and close contact with doctors, nurses, and other health service professionals. In addition to its usefulness to medical social workers and social workers in general, I believe that this book will be helpful to the occupational therapist, physiotherapist, home help organizer, and to all those who work in the voluntary sector at the interface between health and social services. It is more than a dictionary, it is more than a phrase book, although it serves these functions excellently; it is an introduction to the grammar and therefore the culture of the medical world. I believe that its use will promote understanding, increase trade, and reduce the risk of conflict.

J. A. MUIR GRAY, MB, CHB, DPH.
Community Physician,
Oxfordshire Area Health Authority.

Abortion

(Termination of Pregnancy)

The Medical Condition

AGE OF ONSET Any time during child-bearing years.

CAUSE A medical procedure causing the expulsion of the foetus from the womb in the first stages of pregnancy (up to five months). A variety of complications of early pregnancy can cause a spontaneous abortion. This is usually preceded by abdominal pain and vaginal bleeding and occurs in the first three months of pregnancy, but for some women can be a hazard throughout.

COURSE Once pregnancy is established, abortion can be requested under the guidelines of the *Abortion Act 1967*. If it is accepted as necessary, then the earlier it is carried out the less likely is the risk of complications. Very young girls and older women tend to be late in requesting abortion because of ignorance, denial, or conflicting feelings. The initial request is made to the general practitioner, who will normally refer to the hospital gynaecologist for his agreement or refusal to terminate the pregnancy, within the terms of the Act. Abortion can be carried out as an out-patient procedure, but more usually requires admission to hospital. Complications can arise such as bleeding or infection.

EFFECTS For some women termination of pregnancy is a great relief. For others, abortion is a traumatic experience. The decision may have caused great anxiety and conflicting feelings, which often take a long time to resolve. Where there are no medical complications, normal health is quickly restored.

TREATMENT There are three main methods:
(Procedures)

1. Out-patient procedure – prostaglandin pessary – within the first seven weeks.
2. In-patient procedure – the suction method, under general anaesthetic – within the first twelve weeks.
3. In-patient procedure – injection of chemical substance (prostaglandin) to induce a miscarriage artificially – within the first twenty weeks.

Girls under the age of sixteen must have parental consent to any of these procedures.

People Likely to be In Touch

In Hospital Gynaecologist, ward sister, social worker, family planning staff.

At Home General practitioner, health visitor, counselling services (voluntary and statutory), Family Planning Clinic.

Help Needed

There are many reasons for unwanted pregnancy. It can be an expression of unconscious needs, lack of affection, a wish to manipulate, or just a mistake. Whatever the cause, women may need practical help in arranging to see the doctor. Some general practitioners may be reluctant to deal with abortion referrals. Women have the right to ask for prompt help and a second opinion if necessary. Occasionally temporary accommodation either before or after the abortion may be needed. Women need help in understanding the implications of their decision and sometimes support in the face of a rejecting family or boyfriend. Many do not tell their parents. Sometimes it is important to work with the putative father as well. Many women are seen by the hospital social worker at the clinic and it is important to link up with her. Advice on contraceptive methods is given in the hospital or Family Planning Clinics. Help and encouragement to follow this up may be needed.

Resources

The following organizations provide contraceptive advice, pregnancy testing, and abortion counselling
British Pregnancy Advisory Service, (Head Office)
Austy Manor,
Wootton Wawen,
Solihull,
West Midlands B95 6DA.
Telephone Henley-in-Arden (056 42) 3225

Brook Advisory Centre,
233 Tottenham Court Road,
London W1P 9AE.
Telephone 01 580 2991

London Pregnancy Advisory Service,
40 Margaret Street,
London W1.
Telephone 01 409 0281

Release,
1 Elgin Avenue,
London W9.
Telephone 01 603 8564 (24 hour 01 289 1123)

Additional Information

Abortion Act 1967

The Act permits legal abortion if:

1 The continuance of the pregnancy would involve risk to the life of the pregnant woman greater than if the pregnancy were terminated.

2 The continuance of the pregnancy would involve risk of injury to the physical or mental health of the pregnant woman greater than if the pregnancy were terminated.

3 The continuance of the pregnancy would involve risk of injury to the physical or mental health of the existing child(ren) of the family of the pregnant woman greater than if the pregnancy were terminated.

4 There is a substantial risk that if the child were born it would suffer from such physical or mental abnormalities as to be seriously handicapped.

Alcoholism

The Medical Condition

AGE OF ONSET Young adults onwards. Until recently mostly males but females now on the increase.

CAUSE An underlying psychological problem, often coupled with a personality defect. Inability to cope with life and using heavy or habitual drinking as an escape.

COURSE One form may be episodic, with bouts of heavy drinking. The other is steady everyday drinking without severe intoxication. The first drink of the day provides a stimulus to go on drinking, and every fresh situation or problem seems unmanageable without it. The course of the illness depends on the personality and circumstances of the sufferer and his willingness to co-operate with treatment. In chronic cases serious liver disease can develop (cirrhosis) or inflammation of the nerves in legs and arms (peripheral neuritis). Brain damage and even death can result.

EFFECTS It is often extremely hard to tell when someone has become an alcoholic. Increasingly heavy social drinking can be tolerated without much change at first. Irritability and gradual loss of concentration then develop. Later there is total loss of interest, neglect of personal hygiene, and a lack of proper nutrition. Bouts of real drunkenness, 'going on a blind', can last for days or weeks. These bouts may be a response to stress or merely triggered off by the reintroduction to alcohol after abstinence. One specific form of alcoholic mental disturbance is Korsakow's psychosis in which the patient can give an elaborate but entirely illusory description of the day's events. The 'D Ts' (delirium tremens) are bouts of vivid hallucinations in which small furry animals may be seen. If alcohol is withdrawn too rapidly, fits may occur. In cirrhosis of the liver, there is a risk of sudden haemorrhage from the stomach.

TREATMENT The first and most vital aspect of treatment is that the patient should acknowledge the problem. The family, employer, and friends must recognize that he is ill and in need of help. Although he may need 'drying out' in hospital, it is at least as important to give prolonged emotional support to help him to recognize the underlying problems so that he is more able to deal with them. In general, an ex-alcoholic can never safely become a social drinker. Abstinence, even at a late stage, can improve almost all the damaging effects.

People Likely to be In Touch

In Hospital Psychiatrist, Addiction Unit staff, social worker, volunteers – Alcoholics Anonymous.

At Home General practitioner, health visitor, district nurse, Alcoholics Anonymous, community psychiatric nurse.

Help Needed

Community workers often come across this problem as part of work with children and families or with the unemployed and homeless alcoholic man. The illness is usually well established by this stage and unless the patient is ready to face up to the problems, it may only be possible to help alleviate the distress caused to his family. However, social workers should be alert to recognize the problem drinker and seek appropriate help. There is a growing problem of alcoholism amongst women and this can be an equally serious threat to family life. Help will be needed with financial problems, placements and holidays for children, emotional support and counselling. Work should be in close co-operation with medical services – general practitioner, Addiction Unit staff, and Alcoholics Anonymous. When it has become a chronic problem and a man has lost his home and job, it is very difficult indeed to offer appropriate help, unless therapeutic residential accommodation is available. Lonely elderly people may resort to drink for comfort and then neglect themselves.

Resources

Addiction Unit – general practitioner refers to Psychiatrist.

Alcoholics Anonymous, (AA)
7 Moreton Street,
London SW1.
Telephone 01 834 8202
Local groups of Alcoholics Anonymous – support groups for relatives.

National Council on Alcoholism,
Hope House,
45 Great Peter Street,
London SW1P 3LT.
Telephone 01 222 1056

The following organizations provide day and residential care, overnight accommodation for single homeless people, and general advice and help:

National Cyrenians,
13 Wincheap,
Canterbury,
Kent CT1 3TB.
Telephone 0227 51641

Salvation Army International Headquarters,
101 Queen Victoria Street,
London EC4P 4EP.
Information Service –
Telephone 01 236 7020

Richmond Fellowship,
8 Addison Road,
London W14 8DL.
Telephone 01 603 6373
Provides residential therapeutic care.

Voluntary Hostels Association,
33 Longacre,
London WC2.

Health Education Service – see local Health Authority Community Sector.

Amputation

The Medical Condition

AGE OF ONSET Any age.

CAUSE In children and young adults, amputation becomes necessary mostly due to injury caused by accident. Other conditions such as diabetes, gangrene, cancer, or advanced arterial disease (especially in the elderly) can lead to amputation.

COURSE Amputation is a surgical procedure where the wounds of a severed limb are neatly trimmed to a stump. The patient can expect to be in hospital from one to three months depending on his general condition. In the case of accident, the patient is usually in need of intensive hospital care and the amputation can be an emergency measure after great efforts have been made to save the affected limb. In other cases the patient has usually been ill for some time and amputation is the last resort.

EFFECTS Amputation is traumatic, both physically and emotionally. The loss is permanent and the body image is changed. Physical and mental adjustments need to be made to achieve mobility and a new pattern of life. Most amputees do not appreciate the full significance of the loss initially and this is partly due to the fact that the severed nerve endings are still alive and convey messages of pain and other sensations from the lost limb (phantom limb). The amputation of an upper limb is more damaging psychologically and more difficult to replace by an artificial limb. The artificial hand may be more embarrassing than an empty sleeve. Elderly patients may be confined to a wheelchair for the rest of their lives.

TREATMENT After the stump has healed, the patient undergoes rigorous rehabilitation. A temporary limb (pylon) is fitted followed by a permanent limb (prosthesis) two or three months after the operation. The patient attends follow-up appointments at the hospital and at the Artificial Limb and Appliance Centre (ALAC) for some months. Particularly in the younger age groups adaptation to a lost limb can be very successful with a complete resumption of most work and leisure activities.

People Likely to be In Touch

In Hospital Surgeon (orthopaedic or general), specialist in rehabilitation, physiotherapist, social worker, occupational therapist, ALAC staff.

At Home General practitioner, district nurse, health visitor, domiciliary occupational therapist, Disablement Resettlement Officer, school.

Help Needed

Contact with hospital social worker and specialist hospital team is most important. Once the patient is back home there may be problems of suitable housing, employment, and mobility, and work should be in conjunction with the primary health care team. After the special attention in hospital, the patient needs to adjust to his own surroundings. There may be a period of depression and mourning for the lost limb. The family also need to make adjustments and practical and psychological support will be needed. Sexual counselling may be appropriate.

CHECK LIST DHSS Benefits – Mobility Allowance, Attendance Allowance. Home Help. Meals on Wheels. Special Housing. Aids and Adaptations – refer to occupational therapist. Disablement Resettlement Officer – retraining. Car Adaptations. Motability. Day care/hospital/periodic care/holiday/residential care.

Resources

Artificial Limb and Appliance Centre. Regionally based workshops and fitting centres for artificial limbs and wheelchairs. Medical referral required.

British Limbless Ex-Servicemen's Association,
Frankland Moore House,
185-187 High Road,
Chadwell Heath, Essex RM6 6NA.
Telephone 01 590 1124/5.
Local branches advise on pensions, employment, and welfare matters. Runs two convalescent homes. Publishes magazine called *Blesmag*.

Useful addresses:

Bury Boot and Shoe Co. Ltd,
Brandlesholme Road,
Bury, Lancs. (will supply single shoes if required)

Disabled Drivers' Motor Club Ltd,
9 Park Parade,
Gunnersbury Avenue,
London W3 9BD.
Telephone 01 993 6454

See also General Organizations for the Disabled (see page 133).

Ankylosing Spondylitis

The Medical Condition

AGE OF ONSET Young adults, mostly males of athletic habits. There is a hereditary factor.

CAUSE Unknown. It is an arthritic spinal condition.

COURSE Symptoms begin slowly. As the disease progresses there are changes in the bones (vertebrae) of the spine, and they become fused. The disease tends to burn itself out after middle age, but by then there may be some lasting deformity. With treatment, patients can often lead a fairly normal life.

EFFECTS There are recurrent severe episodes of backache and discomfort and sometimes pain in the legs. Symptoms are worse early in the morning. Pain and deformity can arise in various parts of the spine, and the effects of this may radiate out to different parts of the body. Sometimes the spine is permanently deformed, leaving the patient unable to stand erect or to walk normally.

TREATMENT Cortisone type drugs and aspirin are given. Patients must keep as active and mobile as possible between attacks of pain. They should sleep on a firm mattress and practise breathing exercises.

People Likely to be In Touch

In Hospital Rheumatologist, orthopaedic surgeon, physiotherapist, social worker, occupational therapist.

At Home General practitioner, district nurse, domiciliary occupational therapist, Disablement Resettlement Officer.

Help Needed

This disease can hit a young person in their prime when family responsibilities, career, and financial achievements are most important. Loss of mobility and pain may affect employment and leisure activities. Before modern treatment, patients were sometimes left with gross deformity and disability, and these burnt out elderly cases may need assistance at home, help with aids and adaptations, and possibly special nursing or residential care.

CHECK LIST DHSS Benefits – Attendance Allowance. Home Help. Meals on Wheels. Aids and Adaptations – refer to occupational therapist. Disablement Resettlement Officer. Housing. Residential Accommodation for the Elderly.

Resources

National Ankylosing Spondylitis Society,
Honorary Secretary, Mr M. Tanfield,
4 Beaconsfield Road,
Clifton,
Bristol BS8 2TS.
Promotes research and the education and welfare of sufferers.

British Rheumatism and Arthritis Association,
6 Grosvenor Crescent,
London SW1X 7ER.
Telephone 01 235 0902
Advice and information. Caters for welfare needs of members. Runs five specially adapted hotels for use of members. Local Groups.

Arthritis and Rheumatism Council,
Faraday House,
8-10 Charing Cross Road,
London WC2H 0HN.
Telephone 01 240 0871
Fund raising for research only. Publishes quarterly magazine *ARC*. Local branches.

Anorexia Nervosa

The Medical Condition

AGE OF ONSET Adolescence (young women fifteen to twenty-five, rarely young men).

CAUSE Loss of appetite, amounting to rejection of all foods. Thought to be caused by unresolved emotional problems.

COURSE Condition usually noticed first by others. Slowly increasing weakness, frailty, and emaciation. Many recover after several months, some continue to reject food, and up to 10 per cent die.

EFFECTS Severe loss of appetite, restless energy, steady weight loss, failure of menstruation. The patient may be obsessed with special diets. She may eat heartily in company and then withdraw to the toilet to induce vomiting. Severe cases lose their resistance to infections.

TREATMENT Removal to hospital away from the family is often necessary to produce improvement. Drugs, psychotherapy, and behaviour therapy are used, sometimes over a long period.

People Likely to be In Touch

In Hospital General physician, paediatrician, psychiatrist, social worker.

At Home General practitioner, community psychiatric nurse, out-patient psychiatric clinic, day hospital.

Help Needed

Parents and families find it difficult to understand this frightening condition. They feel helpless and inadequate as they watch the disease progress. Their child may be on the brink of death several times. Families may need to take part in psychotherapy, and will need support from community and hospital staff. Some patients find self help groups beneficial. Because of the manipulative nature of some patients with this illness, it is important for all workers concerned to liaise closely and establish patterns of treatment.

Anorexic Aid,
Gravel House,
Copthall Corner,
Chalfont St. Peter,
Bucks.
Telephone Chalfont St Giles 4152
Society for mutual support and fellowship for patients and families.

Arteriosclerotic and Senile Dementia

(Mental Disturbance of the Elderly)

The Medical Condition

AGE OF ONSET Sixty years onwards.

CAUSE Insufficient blood supply to the brain or symptom of advanced age. Arteriosclerosis – hardening of the arteries.

COURSE Gradual onset, possibly after a collapse, faint, or period of speechlessness. Patients show steady deterioration of mental and physical functions, placing great strain on those closest to them. Arteriosclerotic dementia starts earlier and shows more associated physical disability.

EFFECTS Problems of behaviour, memory, judgement, and emotional instability. Physical deterioration, messy habits, wandering night and day. Safety problems, e.g. gas taps and danger of hypothermia.

TREATMENT No cure, but symptoms can be relieved by drugs. Occupational therapy can be helpful. Sometimes nursing care is needed and the patient requires help with all aspects of personal care.

People Likely to be In Touch

In Hospital Psychogeriatrician, geriatrician, neurologist, general physician, hospital social worker, physiotherapist, occupational therapist, psychologist.

At Home General practitioner, community psychiatric nurse, health visitor, district nurse, domiciliary occupational therapist, day hospital/centre, psychiatric hospital team who may be offering short-term relief admissions.

Help Needed

Most people are cared for at home. Assess patient with hospital or primary health care team (general practitioner, health visitor, psychiatric nurse) and identify key workers. Joint planning with family or neighbours/carers to share the burden of caring. Although direct work with patient may be virtually impossible in the accepted sense, continuing regular support and relief for the 'carers' is vital. Programmed admissions to psychogeriatric hospital or residential home throughout the year may postpone or prevent long-term care.

14 **CHECK LIST** DHSS Benefits, e.g. Attendance Allowance, Invalid Care Allowance. Aids and Adaptations – refer to occupational therapist. Home Help. Meals on Wheels. Incontinent Laundry Service. Day care/hospital. Intermittent/permanent residential care. Private nursing home.

Resources

Age Concern England
(National Old People's Welfare Council),
Bernard Sunley House,
60 Pitcairn Road,
Mitcham,
Surrey CR4 3LL.
Telephone 01 640 5431.
Local branch for day centres, clubs, sitters in, visiting, fostering schemes, village van service etc.

National Association for Mental Health (MIND),
22 Harley Street,
London W1N 2ED.
Telephone 01 637 0741.
Specialist advisory body interested in the problems and rights of the mentally ill.

Associations and Charities for the elderly may give financial assistance (see Charities Digest or local directory for voluntary organizations).

Arthritis

The Medical Condition

AGE OF ONSET Can start in teens, but more often in middle to old age.

CAUSE Inflammation of joints due to infection or damage from disease, trauma, and/or the ageing process.

COURSE There are several forms of this disease including gout, but the two most common are:
Rheumatoid Arthritis which may begin at an early age, and is a painful, progressive chronic illness which can lead to severe disability. Two thirds of patients are women.
Osteo-arthritis begins in middle to old age and progresses slowly, causing pain and disability. Where it occurs in certain joints such as the hip, surgery can dramatically alleviate the condition, and therefore the course of the disease. Arthritis is not life threatening.

EFFECTS Pain is the worst feature of this disease, and stiffness of joints, particularly after rest. It may take a very long time to get moving in the morning. Rheumatoid patients can have good and bad spells and are affected by climate. The disease may flare up with stress and eventually cause immobility and deformity.

TREATMENT Drugs are the main source of treatment and some of these have their own side effects. Replacement surgery of certain joints is very effective. Physiotherapy and occupational therapy are used extensively.

People Likely to be In Touch

In Hospital Rheumatologist, orthopaedic surgeon, specialist in rehabilitation, physiotherapist, occupational therapist, social worker.

At Home General practitioner, health visitor, district nurse, home help, hospital out-patients and/or day care, voluntary society.

Help Needed

Where there is a Department of Rheumatology many patients will be known to the hospital social worker. Apart from the disabling effects of the disease, the pain can make the person unable to cope with their normal routine. They may well become irritable and depressed, which has obvious effects on family life. Young married couples may have difficult decisions to make about having children, because of the risk of flare up of the disease. Depending on the degree of disability, there may be sexual problems.

CHECK LIST DHSS Benefits – Attendance Allowance, Mobility Allowance, Disabled Housewives Allowance, Invalid Care Allowance. Motability. Home Help. Meals on Wheels. Employment – Disablement Resettlement Officer. Aids and Adaptations – refer to occupational therapist. Day Care. Periodic/permanent residential care. Holidays. Volunteers.

Resources

British Rheumatism and Arthritis Association,
6 Grosvenor Crescent,
London SW1X 7ER.
Telephone 01 235 0902
Publishes quarterly magazine *Review*. The association administers five hotels, one residential home and a small block of flats. See local groups.

Arthritis and Rheumatism Council,
Faraday House,
8-10 Charing Cross Road,
London WC2H 0HN.
Telephone 01 240 0871
Fund raising for research only. Publishes quarterly magazine *ARC*. See local groups.

General Organizations for the Disabled (see page 133).

Asthma

The Medical Condition

AGE OF ONSET Any age.

CAUSE Asthma is characterized by attacks of difficulty in breathing. These can be caused by allergy, irritation, or infection of the breathing tubes of the lungs. Allergy can be to substances such as pollen, feathers, or food. A hereditary tendency is well recognized, and often it is associated with childhood eczema.

COURSE Acute attacks may be very alarming for patient and family. Difficulty in breathing is usually accompanied by wheezing, cough, and a feeling of constriction of the chest. Attacks can lead to status asthmaticus – one attack merging into another. The disease may subside spontaneously or become chronic.

EFFECTS The majority of sufferers lead normal lives between attacks. With the more severe and chronic conditions the disease may affect the heart and damage the lungs. Many of these people, particularly the elderly, may need hospital admission.

TREATMENT Patients are often referred for allergy tests and this is followed by de-sensitization. Attacks respond dramatically to drugs and inhalations which most people can administer themselves. Very acute attacks may need treatment in Casualty Departments or hospital admission. Physiotherapy and breathing exercises can be helpful. Long-term treatment of chronic asthmatics is difficult and unrewarding. Psychological factors are important and have to be taken into account.

People Likely to be In Touch

In Hospital Paediatrician, chest physician, general physician, allergy clinic, hospital social worker, physiotherapist.

At Home General practitioner, health visitor (could be from Chest Clinic), out-patient clinics, paediatric liaison nurse, school.

Help Needed

Children Not always known to the hospital. Asthma can be a cause of repeated anxiety for children and parents, and help may be needed to prevent over-protection or manipulation of symptoms. It may be helpful to arrange activities outside home. Some children need hospital care and can improve dramatically away from home surroundings. It is important to liaise with social workers on children's units.

Adults Most chronic asthmatics will already be in touch with the hospital. A few may need repeated admissions, and some of these may find it difficult to keep going without this 'crutch'. Chronic asthma should be recognized as a very disabling disease, requiring long-term support. General care and improvement of home environment are important factors.

CHECK LIST DHSS Benefits, e.g. extra heating allowance. Home Help. Meals on Wheels. Aids and Adaptations – refer to occupational therapist. Holidays. Special Schooling. Fares to visit children in hospital – DHSS. Charities.

Resources

Chest, Heart and Stroke Association,
Tavistock House (North),
Tavistock Square,
London WC1H 9JE.
Telephone 01 387 3012
Promotes research and wider knowledge, educational literature, cassettes.

Asthma Research Council,
12 Pembridge Square,
London W2 4EH.
Telephone 01 229 1149
Local Groups. Convalescent and Holiday Homes.

Trade Unions and large industry often have monies or holiday homes of their own.

Autism

The Medical Condition

AGE OF ONSET Birth or during infancy. Boys are affected more than girls.

CAUSE Unknown.

COURSE Autism is a combination of handicaps affecting a child's behaviour and language. The typical autistic child is withdrawn into a private world of his own. Some gradually emerge as more or less normal, but very often they will need a sheltered environment throughout life.

EFFECTS A baby may cry incessantly for hours on end for no apparent reason and nothing his parents can do will comfort him, or he may be unnaturally quiet and unresponsive to pleasure or discomfort and lie quietly disregarding talk, cuddles, attempts to play, etc. The normal mother/child relationship is almost impossible to achieve. Parents feel their love rejected. As the child grows, he is late in talking, picks up meaningless phrases, and the most severe cases may never develop proper speech at all. Some objects seem to hold strange significance and he will stroke them obsessively, smell or taste them. His parents and teachers find him out of reach, remote and preoccupied – often despairing in his isolation. He may become extremely anxious if any of his routines are in the slightest way disturbed. Parting from even the most worthless possessions can cause him great distress. He may be hyperactive and at times utterly reckless of his own safety. It is almost impossible to leave some of these children alone, even for a moment. Some damage themselves considerably by rubbing their skin until it bleeds or by banging their head against a wall, seemingly impervious to pain. Many suffer also from physical handicap or epilepsy. Learning is an immense problem, particularly speech and writing. Some children develop special talents such as unusual skills in music, or in working out mechanical problems.

TREATMENT This is by special education and care throughout childhood and adolescence, mostly on a one-to-one basis. Teaching has to be constant, repetitive, and covering all aspects of the child's life. This may be done at special schools and/or at home. Very disturbed disruptive children and adults are often looked after in special private residential institutions or hospitals for the mentally subnormal because this is the only available resource.

People Likely to be In Touch

In Hospital Paediatrician, psychiatrist, psychologist, social worker, special hospital/school team, paediatric assessment centre.

At Home General practitioner, health visitor, Education Department, local voluntary society.

Help Needed

Parents often react to the child's lack of response by feelings of anxiety, guilt, anger, and despair in their efforts to get through. Some parents totally reject. An autistic child can disrupt a family. In these cases the child will have to be admitted, at least periodically, to institutional care. Social workers will usually be working with the parents. Other members of the family may produce problems as a reaction to the presence of the autistic child.

CHECK LIST DHSS Benefits – Attendance Allowance. Holidays for parents and siblings. Domiciliary occupational therapist for Aids and Adaptations. Self Help Groups for parents. Permanent or periodic care. Baby sitting. Home Help. Voluntary help.

Resources

National Society for Autistic Children,
1a Golders Green Road,
London NW11 8EA.
Telephone 01 458 4375
Provides day and residential centres for care and education. Local groups.

National Society for Mentally Handicapped Children and Adults (MENCAP),
117-123 Golden Lane,
London EC1Y 0RT.
Telephone 01 253 9433
Local branches. Regional Offices. Gateway Clubs for Seniors and Juniors. Residential homes. Welfare visitors.

MIND. National Association for Mental Health,
22 Harley Street,
London W1N 2ED.
Telephone 01 637 0741
See MIND publication – *Children Apart.*

Advisory service. Homes, hostels and boarding schools.

See Helpful Organizations for Handicapped Children (page 136).

Bell's Palsy

The Medical Condition

AGE OF ONSET Adults of any age.

CAUSE Virus infection of the cranial nerve which supplies the muscles of the face.

COURSE Very rapid onset. The patient may even wake up with the condition. In many cases, the virus infection settles quickly and the paralysed muscles recover within a month. If the inflammatory pressure on the nerve continues for longer than this, recovery will take many months, and there may be permanent damage to the face.

EFFECTS The face feels stiff and there may be some pain. The paralysis rapidly develops resulting in a flat, drooped face on one side, with the lower eyelid unable to close properly. These features are characteristic of the condition. There is paralysis of all facial expression on one side, and the patient cannot wrinkle the forehead, close the eye, or smile.

TREATMENT There is no curative treatment. However, the eye needs drops and protection with a shade. Minor surgical procedures are sometimes used to 'hitch up' paralysed muscles.

People Likely to be In Touch

In Hospital Physician, neurologist, neurosurgeon.
At Home General practitioner, district nurse, hospital out-patient follow-up clinic.

Help Needed

Facial disfigurement is a source of great stress and embarrassment. Patients may feel unable to cope with their normal daily routine. Elderly people may need extra help and encouragement at this time, from friends and volunteers.

Resources

Voluntary Agency, e.g. Good Neighbour Scheme.
Age Concern.

Blindness and Partial Sight

The Medical Condition

AGE OF ONSET Any age.

CAUSE Can be congenital, accidental, or the result of various conditions such as cataract, glaucoma, macular degeneration, detached retina, and diabetic retinopathy.

COURSE A minority of children are born blind, but most blindness, with the exception of accidents, develops gradually and poor or absent vision is a condition of old age. Sudden blindness may occur as a result of accident, or for example severe diabetes or a thrombosis near the eye. Prompt diagnosis and treatment can change the course of some conditions and prevent blindness occurring.

EFFECTS Congenital blindness is often associated with other physical and mental handicaps. Sudden blindness is traumatic and changes a person's entire life. The more gradual onset in the elderly gives time for them to adapt but nevertheless can be an extra difficulty when other faculties are failing. Very few people are totally blind and even if registered as such, usually have some residual vision.

TREATMENT Once a person is blind, there is normally little that can be done to restore sight. Partial sightedness can be helped by spectacles, regular checking, and low vision aids. Cataract may be treated by surgery and the supply of very strong spectacles. Glaucoma may be treated by surgery, but more usually with eye drops to delay visual deterioration. Other conditions are treated by surgical procedures, drugs, etc.

People Likely to be In Touch

In Hospital Ophthalmologist, general physician, social worker for the Ophthalmic Unit, Low vision aid clinic.

At Home General practitioner, health visitor, district nurse, mobility and technical officer, County Association for Blind, Education Department, Blind Persons Resettlement Officer – access through Disablement Resettlement Officer.

Help Needed

The Ophthalmologist will send a form (BD 8) to the Social Services Department so that the patient may be included on the Blind and Partially Sighted register if he so wishes. A social worker for the blind or a technical officer should then visit to assess his particular needs. The Local Authority have a responsibility for the training and rehabilitation of the blind. Services include mobility training, teaching of braille and typing, and provision of aids. It may also be necessary to provide residential training for re-orientation or the use of guide dogs. The newly blind may not be ready to accept their condition and will need time before taking advantage of the various services available. Counselling and support will be necessary to help the patient adjust to the loss. Group work can be helpful, particularly for the younger newly blind, and day care and classes play an important part in rehabilitation. Registered patients are entitled to income tax allowances, free radio, reduced television licence fee, and increased supplementary benefit.

CHECK LIST DHSS Benefits. Special allowances for Blind and Partially Sighted. Home Help. Meals on Wheels. Technical Officer. Special Education Department. Blind Persons Resettlement Officer. Voluntary organizations. Clubs. Holidays and outings.

Resources

Royal National Institute for the Blind,
224 Great Portland Street,
London W1N 6AA.
Telephone 01 388 1266
The main source of information on all blind services. Promotes education, training, rehabilitation, employment, and general welfare of all blind people.

County Associations for the Blind run handicraft classes and social clubs, often in conjunction with Social Services Departments, and provide information.

'In Touch' – BBC Radio 4 programme for blind and partially sighted people. Booklet *In Touch* available from the BBC, 35 Marylebone High Street, London W1M 4AA.

Radios and Talking Books available under *Chronically Sick and Disabled Persons Act* – from the Social Services Department.

Brain Tumour

The Medical Condition

AGE OF ONSET Occurs at any age.

CAUSE Unknown. Malignant or non-malignant growth in the brain.

COURSE The tumour causes pressure in the head and may impair the functions of the spinal cord and therefore other functions of the body. It presses upon and may destroy some part of the brain itself, and as it grows larger, symptoms increase. It can be an acute episode responding well to surgery, with return to normal life. Some tumours are inoperable and lead to death. Others, even after operation, leave the patient disabled.

EFFECTS Vary according to position and size of tumour. They may include headache, vomiting, blurred vision, drowsiness and fits. Speech and mental functioning may be impaired.

TREATMENT By surgery and/or radiotherapy, followed by intensive rehabilitation. With inoperable tumours it may only be possible to treat with drugs to reduce the size and pressure in the head.

People Likely to be In Touch

In Hospital Neurologist, neurosurgeon, radiotherapy department, social workers, physiotherapist, occupational therapist.

At Home General practitioner, health visitor, district nurse, hospital out-patient clinics, physiotherapy out-patient clinic, domiciliary occupational therapist.

Help Needed

Liaise closely with hospital social worker and primary health care team. Brain surgery is particularly frightening and patient and family may have fears of mental illness. Patients may be left with long-term disability following surgery or may face distressing deterioration at home and eventual terminal care. Families may need bereavement counselling.

CHECK LIST DHSS Benefits, e.g. Attendance Allowance, Disabled Housewives Allowance. Mobility and Motability. Invalid

Care Allowance. Convalescence/Holiday may be particularly beneficial. Education. Employment – Disablement Resettlement Officer. Aids and Adaptations – refer to occupational therapist. Day Care. Home Help. Meals on Wheels. Voluntary help. Fares for hospital visiting (DHSS or Charities).

Resources

National Society for Cancer Relief,
Michael Sobell House,
30 Dorset Square,
London NW1 5QL.
Telephone 01 402 8125
Will give money for specific purposes or weekly grants for people at home. The Society usually makes a rapid response to requests. They also help to fund a network of terminal care units in conjunction with NHS.

Cancer

(Carcinoma, Sarcoma, Malignancy, Tumour, Growth, 'C.A.' Neoplasm)

The Medical Condition

AGE OF ONSET Any age.

CAUSE Unknown. Probably certain hereditary factors e.g. certain blood groups. Environmental factors include viruses, smoking, X-rays and industrial processes. Almost all the tissues in the body can develop a cancerous growth. This may interfere with adjacent tissues, or spread to other parts of the body through the blood stream (metastases, secondaries).

COURSE The course depends on early diagnosis and treatment. Effective treatment can either cure or slow down the progress of the illness. If there is no treatment, or it is begun too late, the outcome is death. There is a tendency for cancer to be more malignant in young people. In the elderly it may be so benign that it does not materially affect their life expectancy.

EFFECTS These depend on the site of the tumour and response to treatment. Internal cancers are often insidious in the early stages, but may cause weight loss, pain, anaemia, or internal bleeding. The illness may be short or long drawn out.

TREATMENT Drugs, radiotherapy, and surgery. Surgery may sometimes be extensive and mutilating. Radiotherapy and drugs can produce bad side effects and the patient may feel depressed and unwell. In advanced stages of the illness, pain and other symptoms have to be relieved as they arise and specialized nursing may be needed.

People Likely to be In Touch

In Hospital Physician, surgeon, radiotherapist, radiologist, social worker, physiotherapist, occupational therapist.

At Home General practitioner, health visitor, district nurse, radiotherapy out-patients, hospital unit or hospice staff, domiciliary occupational therapist.

Help Needed

Cancer is probably the most feared disease in our society. It is also extremely common and most people will have some involvement with it, if not personally, then with family or friends.

People regard it as a threat to life, although this is by no means always true. It therefore tends to create more anxiety than other equally severe conditions. People who do make a good recovery may need reassurance and encouragement to return to their normal pattern of living. Severe or long term illness can reduce income, and families will need full DHSS benefits, practical aids, and extra money from voluntary organizations. Cancer is still a taboo subject and many people find it difficult to discuss openly. Counselling and psychological support is therefore important for both patient and relatives. Special bereavement counselling may be needed after death. Patients who are dying may need personal help where there is distress and inability to accept the situation. Hospices or Continuing Care Units are available in some areas, and ease the burden by sharing terminal care with relatives. Some relatives may have a sense of failure if the patient is hospitalized during the final stages.

CHECK LIST DHSS Benefits and all special allowances such as diet, heating, etc., Mobility Allowance, and Attendance Allowance. Grants from voluntary societies. Home Help. Night sitting service. Day Care. Intermittent or terminal care, Hospital or Hospice – refer to general practitioner.

Resources

National Society for Cancer Relief,
Michael Sobell House,
30 Dorset Square,
London NW1 6QL.
Telephone 01 402 8125
Will make block grants or weekly allowances for people at home, for relatives visiting hospital, and for holidays. They also fund a network of terminal care units in conjunction with the NHS.

Marie Curie Memorial Foundation,
124 Sloane Street,
London SW1X 9BP.
Telephone 01 730 9157.
Provides nursing homes, night sitters, and nursing services (apply to Community Nursing Officer).

Cruse Clubs. Local and national for widows and widowers.

Welfare benefits from place of employment e.g. Services, G.P.O., British Leyland, etc.

Cancer of the Breast

The Medical Condition

AGE OF ONSET From late twenties to old age. More usual in early to late middle age.

CAUSE See general page on cancer.

COURSE The first sign is either a small lump in the breast, often painless, or a bleeding retracted nipple. The course depends on the promptness of discovery and treatment. Untreated, the disease may spread to other parts of the body, usually with fatal outcome. Treatment can eradicate the cancer entirely. However, there is a fairly high chance of recurrence in later years.

EFFECTS Often none at first, and women may ignore the first symptoms. After surgery normal activity is soon restored, but for some people mental adjustment to the loss of a breast can be very difficult.

TREATMENT Usually surgery (mastectomy) for removal of the breast and sometimes the glands under the arm, often followed by a course of radiotherapy and/or drugs. While still in hospital, patients are fitted with an artificial breast (prosthesis) and special brassiere. They are followed up for several years by the hospital. Some advanced cases are inoperable.

Help Needed

The breast symbolizes femininity, sexual attraction, and motherhood. The loss of a breast is therefore specially significant and healthy adjustment depends on the woman's feelings about herself and her family and social relationships. Counselling may be necessary after discharge from hospital, and husbands also may need help.

Resources

See page 26 on Cancer.

Cancer of the Cervix

The Medical Condition

AGE OF ONSET Adult life. (Less common in unmarried women.)

CAUSE Unknown.

COURSE The cervix (neck of the womb) develops cancerous cells which may lead to a malignant tumour. If it is untreated, the cancer will spread through the pelvic organs and to the rest of the body.

EFFECTS The first symptoms may be slight vaginal discharge, occasionally blood stained, bleeding after intercourse, or excessive menstrual bleeding (menorrhagia).

TREATMENT Usually by surgical removal of the womb (hysterectomy) and radiotherapy (sometimes by implanting radium needles around the cancer site). Patients are followed up for five years. If there is a recurrence, the problems of managing cancer arise.

Prevention Cervical cancer can be detected at a very early stage. When cancerous changes occur in the cervix the disease can remain dormant for some years, and this dormant stage can be detected by examining scrapings of the cervix under a microscope (cervical smears). Women over the age of thirty-five should have a cervical smear every three years. Cervical cytology clinics operate in all areas.

Help Needed

Women are becoming increasingly aware of the need for regular 'screening', although many are still unwilling to attend clinics. Hysterectomy which may be performed for benign tumours as well (fibroids), may come as a great relief for distressing and worrying symptoms. It can however bring feelings of loss, a threat to femininity, and an untimely end to child bearing. Marital and sexual counselling may be necessary.

Resources

See page 26 on Cancer.

Cancer of the Stomach

(Gastric Carcinoma)

The Medical Condition

AGE OF ONSET Middle age and onwards.

CAUSE Unknown. There are sometimes hereditary factors. There may be a past history of other gastric troubles. It is the commonest cause of death from cancer.

COURSE Very variable. Extensive surgery can sometimes be successful, but often gives only temporary benefit, the patient relapsing again later. Death very often occurs within a year.

EFFECTS There is usually dull stomach pain or discomfort, with loss of appetite and weight. Later nausea and vomiting may become persistent.

TREATMENT Early diagnosis and surgery give the only chance of recovery. The whole stomach may have to be removed (total gastrectomy). Inoperable cases will require careful nursing, special diets, and ultimately terminal care.

Help Needed

The relentless progress of this particular cancer is a source of great distress to the onlooking family. There is a continuing need for medical and social support. Community workers liaise with the hospital social worker. Families may need extra practical help if they wish to nurse the patient at home in the terminal stages. Bereavement counselling will usually be needed.

CHECK LIST DHSS Benefits, extra heating, diet allowances. Grants from Voluntary Societies. Liquidizers via Hospital or sometimes under *Chronically Sick and Disabled Persons Act* or voluntary grant. Home Help. Convalescent holiday.

Resources

See page 26 on Cancer.

Cervical Spondylosis

The Medical Condition

AGE OF ONSET Adult life, mainly middle age onwards.

CAUSE Accident, stress, or degenerative changes in neck joints and discs.

COURSE In the early stages there may be painful spasms of the neck muscles, especially when the patient is tired. In more severe cases, the pain can extend into one or both arms, and there may be some wasting in the shoulder muscles 'root symptoms'. Sometimes, especially among elderly people, the spinal cord itself is damaged, and the arms and legs become weak. This state is usually linked with widespread arterial and other disease.

EFFECTS The disease pattern ranges from spasmodic attacks of pain which settle down after a few days or weeks, to extremely severe and chronic disability.

TREATMENT Pain killing drugs and physiotherapy. The wearing of a special collar to ease pain gives support and reduces neck movement. Neck traction (stretching) is sometimes very quickly effective. Rarely is surgery undertaken.

People Likely to be In Touch

In Hospital Neurologist, neurosurgeon, orthopaedic surgeon, consultant in rehabilitation, physiotherapist, occupational therapist, social worker.

At Home General practitioner, district nurse, domiciliary occupational therapist.

Help Needed

Pain and immobility of any kind can affect the practical aspects of life such as employment, housework, driving, leisure activities. They can also have profound effects on mood, personality, and relationships. In middle life, where the condition is spasmodic, there may not be need for much help, except possibly with changing employment or adapting a house so that daily activities do not provoke attacks. Nevertheless pain, and sometimes the need to wear an unsightly collar, does make patients depressed and resentful, or families impatient, and special understanding and counselling may help. Older people with more severe disability may need the whole range of physical and financial aids, and possibly periodic holidays, or even long term residential care.

CHECK LIST DHSS Benefits – Attendance Allowance, Disabled Housewives Allowance. Aids and Adaptations – refer to occupational therapist. Disablement Resettlement Officer. Home Help. Meals on Wheels. Holidays. Day Care. Periodic/permanent residential care.

Resources

General Organizations for the Disabled and Elderly. (See page 133.)

Chronic Bronchitis and Bronchiectasis

The Medical Condition

AGE OF ONSET Usually middle life.

CAUSE Bronchitis is a persistent excretion of mucus from the lungs resulting in productive cough and aggravated by any acute infection (colds, influenza, etc.) or by fumes, and particularly by smoking. Bronchiectasis is more serious and involves distortion and swelling of the bronchial tubes with persistent infection.

COURSE Bronchitis is known as 'The English Disease', and is particularly common in damp and cold climates. It begins with acute attacks and develops into a chronic chest condition, often at its worst in the winter. In the long term the patient may become very disabled and dependent, requiring nursing at home. Sometimes the condition affects the heart.

EFFECTS Persistent cough, expectoration of phlegm, breathlessness on exertion. Disrupts normal pattern of life, particularly employment. Many patients suffer chronic depression.

TREATMENT Cold and damp should be avoided. Acute episodes need antibiotics and soothing remedies such as inhalations. Every crisis tends to be worse than the last. Some patients need oxygen, which they can administer themselves at home. At this stage, they and their families are often aware of a real danger of asphyxia.

People Likely to be In Touch

In Hospital Chest physician, general physician, chest clinic health visitor, social worker, physiotherapist.

At Home General practitioner, health visitor – probably from chest clinic, district nurse, home help, day hospital/centre.

Help Needed

Patients may be referred because of housing and heating problems, particularly where the breadwinner is unemployed because of disability. A good deal of practical help may be needed to support the family because relationship problems often occur. There is a tendency for affected men to be antisocial and many of them live alone. Chest Clinics usually keep in constant touch with patients and will support applications for housing, DHSS Benefits, voluntary grants, etc. Sexual counselling may be necessary.

CHECK LIST DHSS Benefits – Heating, Attendance Allowance, Mobility Allowance, Invalid Care Allowance. Housing. Employment – Disablement Resettlement Officer. Aids and Adaptations – refer to occupational therapist. Day Care. Holidays. Voluntary Grants. Residential Care permanent/temporary. Convalescence. Public Employers and Union Grants.

Resources

Chest, Heart and Stroke Association,
Tavistock House (North),
Tavistock Square,
London WC1H 9JE.
Telephone 01 387 3012
Promotes research and wider knowledge, educational literature, cassettes.

Convalescent and Holiday Homes – Trade Unions and large industry often have monies and holiday/convalescent homes of their own.

Coeliac Disease

(Gluten-Enteropathy or Sprue Syndrome)

The Medical Condition

AGE OF ONSET Childhood, after weaning. More girls than boys.

CAUSE An inability of the gut to absorb food properly. This is caused by an inflammation of the internal lining of the gut due to an allergic reaction to gluten.
Gluten is the main protein of starchy foods derived from wheat, rye, barley, and oats. It is not present in rice and other selected starches.

COURSE The entire condition is reversed by eliminating gluten from the diet. Unfortunately, starchy foods are so readily available that relapses are common. The condition is usually more easily controlled in adults.

EFFECTS The child shows all the signs of malnutrition, i.e. thin wasted limbs, sparse hair, listlessness, etc. They have a distended abdomen and frequent offensive bowel motions. They may well be over-protected by anxious parents and commonly emerge as bright, difficult, and self-centred children.

TREATMENT Gluten free diet is necessary for life. It is more than likely that the child will be taken into hospital initially.

People Likely to be In Touch

In Hospital Paediatrician, dietician, social worker to the paediatric unit, ward sister.
At Home General practitioner, health visitor.

Help Needed

Work should be in close liaison with staff of paediatric clinic and health visitor. In the early stages of the disease, when the child is failing to thrive and irritable, parents' anxiety will be high. If, in addition, social conditions and parental care are poor, long-term support may be necessary until the family have become accustomed to the condition.

CHECK LIST If family in receipt of Supplementary Benefit – special allowance for diet.

Financial help may be available from charities. See Helpful Organizations for Children (page 136).

Colostomy and Ileostomy

The Medical Condition

AGE OF ONSET Any age.

CAUSE Severe bowel disease or congenital conditions requiring surgical intervention. An artificial opening is made in the abdominal wall through which the bowel contents discharge. This is known as a stoma. The most common indication in older people is cancer of the bowel, in younger people, ulcerative colitis (see page 126).

COURSE The decision to operate may follow a long illness but emergency surgery may be necessary. The stoma is sometimes closed after a period of weeks or months, allowing bowel function to return to normal. Some however are permanent and must then become part of normal life.

EFFECTS After the operation the patient has to learn to live with this unnatural orifice at the front of his body. Those who have had long-term problems may view the operation as a welcome relief. Most patients have anxieties about smell, effect on relationships, clothing, loss of libido and body image, and disposal of waste.

TREATMENT A small disposable bag is strapped to the abdomen around the stoma, which the patient learns to change himself. The hospital team provide counselling and practical teaching on management of the stoma. Diet is important and patients learn gradually to recognize foods which cause discomfort or affect the discharge. A variety of adhesives and creams are available to care for the skin around the stoma. Most large hospitals have a stoma sister who sees patients at clinic and follows up with home visits. Some patients learn to irrigate the stoma as an alternative to using a bag, but this method is not in general use.

People Likely to be In Touch

In Hospital Surgeon, physician, social worker, stoma sister.

At Home General practitioner, hospital out-patient clinic, district nurse, stoma sister, volunteer from Ileostomy Association.

Help Needed

Stoma surgery usually follows illness which has been life threatening or extremely debilitating. Families may need counselling and guidance. Initially many people regard the stoma with great distaste. Sometimes it is helpful for patients to meet others who have made a successful adjustment. It is important to liaise with the hospital team, stoma sister, and primary health-care team. Patients should be encouraged to exploit the humorous side of minor embarrassments and to lead a normal and active life. Sexual counselling may be needed.

CHECK LIST DHSS Benefits. Convalescence/recuperative holidays.

Resources

Ileostomy Association of Great Britain and Northern Ireland,
23 Winchester Road,
Basingstoke,
Hampshire RG21 1UE.
Telephone Basingstoke 21288
Local Branches – give advice and help to patients about to or who have just had surgery. Hospital and home visiting organized.

Colostomy Welfare Group,
38/39 Eccleston Square,
London SW1V 1PB.
Telephone 01 828 5175
Consultation, advice, and help for patients.

Congenital Dislocation of the Hip

(CDH)

The Medical Condition

AGE OF ONSET At birth. Girls affected more than boys.

CAUSE Unknown. The socket in the pelvis is too shallow to hold the head of the femur (long bone in the leg). This means that the hip joint may easily dislocate or may already be dislocated at birth.

COURSE Usually diagnosed soon after birth. Early treatment and correction will allow normal formation of the joint. If diagnosis and treatment are delayed, more complex measures are necessary, but most children achieve symptom free walking. There is a risk of osteoarthritis in later life.

EFFECTS If untreated at an early stage, walking is delayed and the child walks with a dipping limp. In approximately one third of children both hips are affected.

TREATMENT Methods vary according to the age of the child. Babies under six months are immobilized and the joints corrected by splints or plaster cast. Older children are treated in hospital by traction (stretching), surgery, and correction in plaster. Hospital care alternates with periods at home. Screening for this condition is carried out in maternity hospitals and post natal clinics.

People Likely to be In Touch

In Hospital Paediatrician, orthopaedic surgeon, social worker, physiotherapist.

At Home General practitioner, health visitor.

Help Needed

This condition can be very distressing for a new mother. Fortunately, much reassurance can be given about a successful outcome. Nevertheless, for babies in splints and needing intermittent hospital care there may be problems in establishing feeding, sleeping, and the normal bonding with the mother. Parents may have difficulty in visiting hospital from long distances or in coping with other children. Some will need accommodation in or near the hospital, and extra financial help.

Workers should liaise closely with hospital and primary health care team.

CHECK LIST DHSS Benefits – fares for visiting hospital. Temporary Foster Home. Family aide. Daily minder. Home Help. Voluntary help.

Resources

See Helpful Organizations for Children (page 136) for visiting and other expenses.

Crohn's Disease

The Medical Condition

AGE OF ONSET Usually between fifteen and thirty-five years.

CAUSE This is an inflammatory condition of the bowel. The cause is not clearly understood.

COURSE The disease follows a relapsing and remitting course over many years. Patients may never feel quite well and usually need to curtail their activities. The outlook varies. Some make a complete recovery after treatment, but a proportion become chronic invalids.

EFFECTS The abdomen is distended and painful, and attacks can be mistaken for acute appendicitis. These systems are associated with either constipation or diarrhoea. The disease attacks the gut, sometimes causing the formation of abscesses which work their way through to the skin (fistulae) and there can also be bowel obstruction. Patients may show signs of malnutrition and suffer from depression.

TREATMENT By drugs, and often surgery to remove affected parts of the bowel. In some cases repeated surgery is necessary, and the patient may be left with a colostomy or ileostomy. (See page 37.)

People Likely to be In Touch

In Hospital Physician and surgeon, social worker.
At Home General practitioner, health visitor, district nurse.

Help Needed

Work with hospital and primary health care team. Crohns is a worrying disease to patient and family, and there may be hidden fear of cancer. Frequent admissions to hospital disrupt family life and employment, and long term social work support may be needed.

CHECK LIST DHSS Benefits. Holidays for patient and family. Convalescence. Home Help.

Resources

There are no specific resources.
See ileostomy/colostomy (page 37).

Cystic Fibrosis

(Fibrocystic Disease or Mucoviscidosis)

The Medical Condition

AGE OF ONSET Birth.

CAUSE A hereditary condition characterized by changes in the pancreas, lungs, intestines, and mucus secreting glands. Both parents carry the affected genes, but do not show signs of the disease.

COURSE The affected child fails to thrive from infancy. Parents bring up the children in a background of chronic ill health, and repeated acute crises, often needing admission to hospital. Despite improved treatment, this is a life-threatening condition. Few children survive to adult life, and rarely to old age. Death usually occurs due to chest complications.

EFFECTS Symptoms appear soon after birth. The baby is emaciated despite a good appetite, the abdomen is distended, diarrhoea is common, and a chronic cough is present which often develops into pneumonia. The consistency of the mucus in the respiratory and digestive passages is abnormal, reducing their efficiency. Digestion of food is interfered with and the child is forever trying to clear thickened mucus from the lungs. Abscesses and fibrous tissue may form in the lungs. The ailing child may become hypochondriacal and manipulative, but in spite of the difficulties, may be intellectually able.

TREATMENT In the last few years, earlier diagnosis, new forms of treatment, and better management in special units, have improved the chance of survival. Diet control, drugs, and physiotherapy are used. This may entail much out-patient supervision, and quite complicated regimes for the parents and child.

People Likely to be In Touch

In Hospital Paediatrician, physician, chest physician, dietician, social worker for paediatric unit, physiotherapist.

At Home General practitioner, health visitor, district nurse, special education department, domiciliary physiotherapist, chest clinic staff, hospital out-patient clinic.

Help Needed

Liaise closely with hospital social worker and primary health-care team. Families will need practical and emotional help over a long period. It may be that parents and child will get their help from the hospital team, but other siblings may suffer and need help in their own right. Hospital and community workers should plan together to ensure appropriate support for the family. Bereavement counselling may be necessary.

CHECK LIST DHSS Benefit – Attendance Allowance, Extra Heating, Diet Allowance, Family Income Supplement. Home Help. Child minder. Voluntary help. Holidays.

Resources

Cystic Fibrosis Research Trust,
5 Blyth Road,
Bromley,
Kent BR1 3RS.
Telephone 01 464 7211
Finances research, helps and advises patients. Holiday caravans for hire at reasonable cost.
Local groups.

See list of Helpful Organizations for Handicapped Children, e.g. The Family Fund (page 138).

Deafness

The Medical Condition

AGE OF ONSET Birth onwards.

CAUSE Congenital deafness may be due to pregnancy complications, birth injury, hereditary factors, ear malformation, or disease. Acquired deafness can be due to a variety of diseases, injury to the ear or head, prolonged exposure to loud noise, or the side effects of drugs.

COURSE This varies, depending on the cause. It ranges from a sudden traumatic cut off to a gradual deterioration of the hearing over many years.

EFFECTS Congenital deafness hinders all areas of the child's development – intellectual, speech, language, personality, and sometimes the physical well being. It can be associated with other physical and mental handicaps. Communication remains a difficulty throughout life. Many people have intermittent or continuous loud noises in the head (tinnitus) or have a balance disorder (see entry on Ménières Disease). Deafness can affect a person's whole outlook on life and personality traits can become exaggerated. Because of their isolation and lack of social intercourse, they may appear to be egocentric. There is often an underlying depression which can be missed. With age, most people become deaf to some degree and this can proceed to total deafness.

TREATMENT Sometimes deafness can be treated by surgery and/or a variety of hearing aids. Drugs are used to treat ear disease. Patients needing a hearing aid should *always* consult their general practitioner, who will refer them for proper assessment at the local hospital Ear, Nose and Throat Department.

People Likely to be In Touch

In Hospital Ear, Nose and Throat Consultant, hearing therapist, hearing aid department, social worker, Paediatric Assessment Centre.

At Home General practitioner, health visitor (tests all babies' hearing at one to five years), school medical service, peripatetic teachers of the deaf (Education Department), specialist social worker.

Help Needed

Liaise with specialist social worker for the deaf, who will be working with a voluntary agency or local authority. Usually they will deal with all pre-lingually deaf patients and will advise on others. With deaf children, the hearing therapist and special teacher are very significant people to both the child and the parents. It may be necessary to establish the key worker. Children are assessed annually at the Ear, Nose and Throat Department or school audiology clinics. Workers should ask to be present or submit a report. Communication is the main problem arising from deafness and the frustration and inability to express themselves can lead to behavioural problems. In adults, particularly the elderly, deafness can become another isolating factor, even if they are not living alone. Social work for the deaf will assist with finding work for deaf patients and introduce them to their new jobs.

Resources

Some areas will have a social centre providing recreational facilities, lip reading classes, sign language courses, and a specialist social work team.

Aids such as visual door bells, alarms, listening devices – available under *Chronically Sick and Disabled Persons Act 1970* from Social Services Departments.

Many private hearing aids are available. Patients wishing to purchase these should always be advised by their general practitioner and Ear Nose and Throat Specialist on the best type for their particular problem.

Royal National Institute for the Deaf,
105 Gower Street,
London WC1E 6AH.
Telephone 01 387 8033
Comprehensive service for the deaf. Residential establishments such as schools and training centres.

British Deaf Association,
38 Victoria Place,
Carlisle CA1 1HU.
Telephone Carlisle 20188
Primarily concerned with promoting the welfare of profoundly deaf people. Provides information on social clubs and welfare services.

British Association of the Hard of Hearing,
6 Great James Street,
London WC1N 3DA.
Telephone 01 405 5182
Promotes formation of local groups and social activities for the hard of hearing. Gives advice on all hearing problems.

National Deaf Children's Society,
31 Gloucester Place,
London W1H 4EA.
Telephone 01 486 3251
Provides information services on all matters concerning deaf children and their welfare.

Breakthrough Trust,
Charles W. Gillett Centre,
Selly Oak Colleges,
Birmingham B29 6LE.
Telephone 021 472 6447
Breakthrough seeks to integrate deaf and hearing children and adults. Has a number of regional and local groups.

Depression

(Neurotic and Reactive)

The Medical Condition

AGE OF ONSET Mainly adolescence onwards.

CAUSE Reactive depression is a reaction to an abnormality or change in life pattern. Neurotic depression occurs in people who have made abnormal adjustments to life prior to the depression.

COURSE Often begins insidiously and may last for weeks or months. There is usually a return to normal health with or without treatment, but the condition may recur.

EFFECTS There is a loss of vitality, interest, and sexual drive, a feeling of sadness, and an inability to carry on with normal life. The patient has difficulty getting to sleep and appetite can be affected. Sometimes depression is accompanied by anxiety and the patient will be agitated, hand wringing, indecisive, perspiring, and have a faster than normal heart beat.

TREATMENT Usually treated with anti-depressant drugs and mild sedatives. Some patients however come through on their own or with the counselling support of the doctor, social worker, or friend, etc.

People Likely to be In Touch

In Hospital Psychiatric team, doctor, nurse, occupational therapist, social worker.

At Home General practitioner.

Help Needed

Counselling on its own can help some patients. With this type of depression patients are still in touch with reality and they can be helped to understand the reason for their condition. Patients will need consistent and reliable help. It is important to work closely with the general practitioner and psychiatric team if they are involved. Relatives will also need support and family therapy may be appropriate.

CHECK LIST DHSS Benefits. Home Help. Voluntary Visitors. Social activities.

National Association for Mental Health (MIND),
22 Harley Street,
London W1N 2ED.
Telephone 01 637 0741
Advisory service and local group activities.

CRUSE,
Cruse House,
126 Sheen Road,
Richmond,
Surrey TW9 2DF.
Telephone 01 940 2660
Organization for widows and widowers and their children. Local branches offer advice, counselling, and social activities.

Samaritans,
17 Uxbridge Road,
Slough,
Bucks SL1 1SN.
Telephone Slough 32713.
Local emergency services for those feeling suicidal or lonely.

Depression

(Psychotic, Endogenous)

The Medical Condition

AGE OF ONSET Throughout life span.

CAUSE Inherited tendency. Endogenous means 'coming from the inside' rather than the external factors surrounding the patient.

COURSE The course depends on early diagnosis and availability of treatment. If untreated, the depression can last for weeks, months, or even years, and there is a real risk of suicide. With treatment there is a return to normal, but the condition is likely to recur.

EFFECTS Initially there is a general slowing down of all mental and physical activity, which can in severe cases progress to a state of stupor. There is a feeling of total misery and hopelessness, reduction in appetite, loss of interest in work, self, and sexual activity. Sleep is disturbed and patients waken early in the morning which is their worst time of day. Some indulge in aimless activity, fidgeting and wandering about in an agitated state. Some patients swing from depression to a manic state (manic-depressive psychosis). The mood swings can fluctuate quickly or over long periods. Some women develop depression after childbirth (puerperal depression).

TREATMENT Patients are normally referred to the psychiatric department. Anti-depressant drugs are used and sometimes ECT (electro-convulsive therapy). Drugs such as Lithium are used to regulate mood swings in manic depressive states. Symptoms and behaviour are closely monitored and group or psychotherapy is sometimes used. With appropriate treatment, most women with puerperal depression make a good recovery, although the condition is likely to recur with subsequent births.

People Likely to be In Touch

In Hospital Psychiatric team, doctor, nurse, occupational therapist, social worker.

At Home General practitioner, community psychiatric nurse, voluntary organizations, day centre/hospital.

Help Needed

Work with these patients in the community involves supporting families during the illness, co-operating with the hospital team in the rehabilitation programme, and recognizing and reporting signs of relapse. Many patients with these types of depression will need long term support, and relatives will be anxious about the real risk of suicide. Recurring depression and the inaccessibility of the patient tends to wear down even the most caring family.

CHECK LIST DHSS Benefits. Home Help. Voluntary Visitors. Day Care/Hospital. Hostel/residential care. Holidays for patient and family.

Resources

National Association for Mental Health (MIND),
22 Harley Street,
London W1N 2ED.
Telephone 01 637 0741
Advisory Service. Runs several homes and hostels. Bi-monthly magazine *Mind Out.*

Mental After-Care Association,
Eagle House,
110 Jermyn Street,
London SW1Y 6HB.
Telephone 01 839 5953
Hostels for rehabilitation after discharge from hospital and homes for long term care. Recuperative holiday accommodation.

Samaritans,
17 Uxbridge Road,
Slough,
Bucks SL1 1SN.
Telephone Slough 32713
Local emergency services for those feeling suicidal and lonely.

Richmond Fellowship,
8 Addison Road,
London W14 8DL.
Telephone 01 603 6373
Residential short and long term therapeutic care.

Diabetes

The Medical Condition

AGE OF ONSET Any age. More common after middle age.

CAUSE A malfunctioning of the pancreas (which produces insulin). Can be hereditary. Obesity is a contributory factor.

COURSE Often discovered by accident during tests for other illnesses. Nowadays most diabetics are well controlled, and although their longevity is slightly below average, most of them can lead a fairly normal life.

EFFECTS Initially thirst, increased urinary output, and a tendency to coma. In long standing diabetes, heart disease, kidney disorders, blindness, and gangrene may result.

TREATMENT The disease can often be controlled by diet, and patients will receive guidance from the hospital dietician or general practitioner. In more severe cases, patients are taught to test their urine daily, and to self-administer insulin by injection to balance their blood sugar. This daily routine calls for self discipline and, to a certain extent, an ordered life. Patients are taught to recognize their own symptoms of imbalance and compensate accordingly.

COMA *Hypoglycaemia* caused by overdose of insulin or delay in taking food after injection, or excessive exercise. Rapid onset. Treatment – administering sugar or glucose.
Hyperglycaemia caused by delay in giving injections, or an overindulgence in high calorie food. Slow onset. Treatment – giving insulin or drugs.

People Likely to be In Touch

In Hospital General physician (diabetic clinic), paediatrician, dietician, psychiatrist, hospital social worker. Patient may be involved in therapeutic groups.

At Home General practitioner, district nurse, health visitor, sometimes special diabetic nurse from the hospital, school, Education Department, domiciliary occupational therapist.

Help Needed

Workers are likely to come across the more long standing cases who may be handicapped through blindness or amputation.

These patients will almost certainly be known to the social worker of the diabetic clinic in hospital. Parents with diabetic children may need help in allowing them independence. People living alone, with severe social problems and with manipulative or self destructive impulses, will need help. Patients should be assessed in close co-operation with general practitioner and hospital staff. There may be cases where it will be appropriate to ask for a psychiatric opinion.

CHECK LIST If in receipt of Supplementary Benefit – special allowance for diet. For the more elderly and disabled – Home Help, Meals on Wheels (diets). Aids and Adaptations – refer to occupational therapist. Services for the blind (see page 23).

Resources

British Diabetic Association,
10 Queen Anne Street,
London W1M 0BD.
Telephone 01 323 1531
Provides information and advice. Organizes children's holidays, also education cruises and holidays abroad. Bi-monthly newspaper – free to members – called *Balance,* plus cassettes for registered blind.

Chemists offer a range of diabetic foods.

Local Diabetic Association may organize self help groups.

Drug Dependence

The Medical Condition

AGE OF ONSET Any age. Usually adolescence.

CAUSE Regular intake of certain drugs until the patient becomes dependent upon them. Can be a response to social and family pressures, and some personality types are more liable to addiction than others.

COURSE Dependence may start insidiously. The course depends on whether the patient seeks treatment and can resettle afterwards into life without drugs. If so, he can be helped, but the relapse rate is very high indeed. If he does not seek or respond to treatment he may steadily deteriorate mentally and physically. The outcome is sometimes death.

EFFECTS Cocaine and the amphetamines are alerting and exhilarating, morphine and heroin (the latter the most dangerous) bring optimism and relaxation, barbiturates and sedatives sleep. Heroin is given by injection and is often mixed with barbiturates or other substances. Cannabis and related drugs are less physiologically addictive but can produce mental damage. Interest in normal life is reduced and values changed. Addicts often live in fear that their drug supplies will run out and may go to extreme lengths to prevent this. Personal hygiene and nutrition are neglected and there is increased vulnerability to infections and other illnesses. Injection sites can become infected by the use of dirty syringes and needles.

TREATMENT By withdrawal of drugs in hospital or special unit. Withdrawal symptoms may be very severe, but it is usually possible to achieve temporary success with even the most dangerous drugs. The more critical part of treatment is resettlement into normal life in the community. Counselling or group therapy may be needed over a long period.

People Likely to be In Touch

In Hospital Staff of psychiatric hospital or drug addiction unit (psychiatrist, psychologist, nursing staff, occupational therapist, social worker).

At Home General practitioner, community psychiatric nurse, hospital or unit staff.

Help Needed

Drug addiction may present as one of a range of adolescent/family problems. Referral may come via the police. It is important to work closely with the general practitioner and the hospital or unit staff. Drug taking is a response to the stress of daily living, and anything that alters the conscious state is a relief. Drugs are expensive and in order to maintain the supply addicts may turn to crime, such as breaking into chemists' shops and hospital pharmacies, or stealing money in order to pay 'pushers'. They may become involved in 'drug rings'. Life can be disordered and disorganized, sometimes on the move, and everything becomes subject to the availability of the drug. Social workers may need to work with relatives while the unit supports the addict, and later, help through the period of adjustment to normal life.

Resources

Standing Conference on Drug Abuse,
125 Kennington Park Road,
London SE11.
Gives information on Regional Drug Addiction Units.

Association for the Prevention of Addiction,
9 St James Street,
Covent Garden,
London WC2.
Telephone 01 836 3781

Directory of Projects – Published by National Association for the Care and Resettlement of Offenders.

Eczema

The Medical Condition

AGE OF ONSET Any age.

CAUSE Many causes, including inherited predisposition, allergy to certain substances or foods, external irritants, and probably a strong emotional factor.

COURSE Eczema is a form of dermatitis and there are several different types. The course and outlook are uncertain because of the individual combination of factors involved. If the causal problems can be dealt with, there is a reasonable chance of a cure. Where this is not possible the outlook is poor and the disease may lapse into a chronic state.

Infantile Eczema. Quite young babies can develop eczema and this seems more difficult to control where the mother/child relationship is unsatisfactory. The condition may clear up when the child feels more independent, but may recur in adolescence.

EFFECTS May occur on any part of the body. The skin reddens and can develop blisters. If the condition becomes chronic there is a thickening of the skin. There is extreme itching and an intense desire to scratch, which is difficult to deal with in small children. Adults prone to leg ulcers can develop eczema in the same area.

TREATMENT Once the cause is identified, steps are taken to alleviate or remove it. Drugs are given and ointments applied to the affected areas. Hospital admission may be necessary in some cases.

People Likely to be In Touch

In Hospital Dermatologist, paediatrician, psychiatrist, social worker.

At Home General practitioner, district nurse, health visitor, Disablement Resettlement Officer.

Help Needed

This disease may be a component of wider social and emotional problems. Distress can be caused by the unsightly patches on the skin. Help may be needed in changing the patient's home or work environment, and counselling for stress in family or personal relationships.

Resources

National Eczema Society,
5-7 Tavistock Place,
London WC1H 9SR.
Telephone 01 388 4097
Provides education and information services. Aims to increase understanding through local self help groups.

Epilepsy

The Medical Condition

AGE OF ONSET Childhood or later years.

CAUSE Epilepsy may be caused by brain abnormality or brain damage which may occur by accident, tumour or effects of surgery. Normally however it is 'idiopathic', i.e. no abnormality can be found in the brain.

COURSE *Petit mal* A mild form of epilepsy which starts in childhood or adolescence and is characterized by momentary loss of consciousness without convulsions. Sometimes difficult to detect and not necessarily disabling. Very rarely continues into adult life.

Grand Mal Classically a major fit starts abruptly with loss of consciousness or a short warning or 'aura'. The body becomes rigid with jerking movements of the limbs, heavy breathing, clenched teeth and sometimes incontinence of urine. The person then relaxes and passes into coma and then deep sleep. The features vary from person to person.

EFFECTS There is still a good deal of stigma and folk lore surrounding epilepsy. Many epileptic people are perfectly normal except during a fit. Nevertheless, the long term effects of severe and frequent fits and the need for high dosage of drugs, does eventually appear to affect personality. Epileptics have difficulty in finding employment because of people's fear of fits and the danger of self damage by machinery, etc. They are not allowed to drive, unless they have been free of fits for three years, even though they are controlled by drugs. (The restrictions are less strict when fits occur only at night.)

TREATMENT Fits are controlled by drugs and patients often need admission to hospital to establish the correct dosage. Rarely, surgery may help. Psychiatric help is often needed for patients with personality disorders.

People Likely to be In Touch

In Hospital Neurologist, general physician, paediatrician, psychiatrist, psychologist, social worker, occupational therapist.

At Home General practitioner, health visitor, domiciliary occupational therapist, school, special education department, Disablement Resettlement Officer, hospital out-patient clinics, adult training centres, sheltered workshops.

Children need careful surveillance of drug regime by general practitioner and hospital as needs change. Parents may need help in accepting the condition and in management of milestones, such as school and first employment. Children are very often 'labelled' and restricted by the attitudes of staff and peers. For example, they may be prevented from playing energetic games or swimming, which isolates them and handicaps normal development. Social workers need to co-ordinate the efforts of health, education, and social services.

Adults Most epileptics who are referred to social services have chronic problems relating to employment, family relationships, community relationships, housing and transport. Very often the patient needs support and advice in acceptance and management of their epilepsy. This can only be achieved by co-operation with the general practitioner and/or the hospital team.

CHECK LIST Disablement Resettlement Officer – retraining. Sheltered Workshops etc. Hostel Accommodation.

Resources

British Epilepsy Association,
Crowthorne House,
New Wokingham Road,
Wokingham,
Berkshire RG11 3AY.
Telephone Crowthorne (03446) 3122
Helps and advises people, provides information service. Addresses of local Action for Epilepsy Groups available from British Epilepsy Association.

Voluntary Hostel Association,
33 Longacre,
London WC2.
Placements – Telephone 01 836 0193

National Association for Mental Health (MIND),
22 Harley Street,
London W1N 2ED.
Telephone 01 637 0741
Specialist advisory body interested in the problems and rights of the mentally ill.

Richmond Fellowship,
8 Addison Road,
London W14 8DL.
Telephone 01 603 6373
Provides residential care if epilepsy is controlled.

Friedreich's Ataxia

The Medical Condition

AGE OF ONSET Childhood and adolescence.

CAUSE Inherited disease of the nervous system which may affect several members of the same family.

COURSE Gradual onset, steadily progressive distressing disability. Does not appreciably shorten life, so very prolonged invalidity is common. The earlier the onset, the worse the outcome.

EFFECTS Clumsiness, reeling walk, speech difficulty, poor eyesight, weakening muscles, loss of posture. The combination of these disabilities makes communication and social life extremely difficult. There may be emotional instability with temper tantrums.

TREATMENT No curative treatment is known. Sometimes possible to control symptoms, i.e. drugs for tremor, splints for limbs. Genetic counselling may be advisable.

People Likely to be In Touch

In Hospital Neurologist, general physician, speech therapist, physiotherapist, occupational therapist, social worker.

At Home General practitioner, health visitor, domiciliary occupation therapist, day centre/hospital, sheltered workshop, school social worker.

Help Needed

Normally the effects of the disease become disabling just as the child reaches adolescence. His whole social, intellectual and physical development is affected. He and his family will need advice, help, and services from that time on. There will be particular stress and anxiety if more than one member is affected. In some cases, care in a Young Disabled Unit or other institution may be the best solution. Sexual counselling may be necessary.

CHECK LIST DHSS Benefits – Attendance Allowance, Mobility Allowance. Aids and Adaptations – refer to occupational therapist. Housing. Education. Employment. Home Help. Meals on Wheels. Day Care. Periodic/Permanent Residential Care. Holidays. Voluntary help.

Friedreich's Ataxia Group,
Bolsover House,
5-6 Clipstone Street,
London W1.
Telephone 01 636 2042
Sponsors research and provides assistance and advice to patients and families.

General Organizations for the Disabled (see page 133).

Haemophilia

The Medical Condition

AGE OF ONSET Birth.

CAUSE Inherited condition affecting only males. The defect is carried by the mother, and an affected male cannot pass the defect to his sons. Therefore, the disease always skips a generation. Blood clotting is abnormally delayed and sufferers can bleed excessively from trivial wounds and also internally into muscles and joints.

COURSE Haemophilia is a constant factor to be lived with. Patients necessarily lead a protected existence. It is a life threatening condition and can lead to permanent disability.

EFFECTS Severe pain is often associated with bleeds. Muscles and joints can be so badly damaged that permanent disability may follow. It is easy for the patient to become self-centred, demanding, and manipulative.

TREATMENT Certain hospitals are designated as Haemophilia Centres. Treatment is by plasma transfusion and drugs and immobilization of damaged joints. Genetic counselling of family is necessary. When the child reaches seven years, parents can be taught to use drugs and treat their children at home for minor bleeds.

People Likely to be In Touch

In Hospital Hospital designated as Regional Centre. Haematologist, orthopaedic surgeon, physiotherapist, social worker.

At Home General practitioner, but continuous involvement with hospital centre more likely. Patients can get help and advice from centre (usually a 24-hour service). Domiciliary occupational therapist.

Help Needed

The majority of help is given by the staff at the Haemophilia Centre. The hospital social worker may ask for support for patients living long distances from the Centre. School and employment are affected and parents almost inevitably feel guilty and over-anxious.

NB. There can be confusion between children suspected of

non-accidental injury and children with bruises from an internal bleed.

CHECK LIST DHSS Benefits – hospital fares, Attendance, Mobility Allowance, Invalid Care Allowance. Employment – Disablement Resettlement Officer. Housing. Education. Aids and Adaptations – refer to occupational therapist. Home Help. Holidays. Residential care.

Resources

The Haemophilia Society,
PO Box 9,
16 Trinity Street,
London SW1 1DE.
Telephone 01 407 1010
Can give grants and loans and provides advice and information. Local groups provide social activities and raise funds.

General Organizations for the Disabled (see page 133).

Voluntary Hostels Association,
33 Longacre,
London WC2.
Placements – Telephone 01 836 0193

Heart Block

(Pacemakers)

The Medical Condition

AGE OF ONSET Occasionally in childhood, but more commonly in middle to old age.

CAUSE The normal heart has the ability to relax and contract rhythmically, keeping the pace at about seventy to eighty beats per minute. The 'pacemaking' function is set at about the point where the big blood vessels enter the heart. Failure of this function causes heart block. In children, the condition is caused by congenital abnormality of the heart and in adults by a degenerative disease of the coronary arteries or the heart muscle itself.

COURSE The patient shows signs of acute heart failure and debility. It is then noticed that the pulse is very slow (forty or less per minute). Once an artificial pacemaker is inserted the patient should return to relatively normal health.

EFFECTS This slow heart rate can result in fainting attacks, debility, and poor mental function, and the whole of life is therefore adversely affected.

TREATMENT Artificial pacemakers can be inserted surgically. The pacemaker delivers tiny intermittent electric shocks to the heart muscle, stimulating contractions at the normal rate. These devices are now extremely reliable and seldom go wrong. Recharging is a quarterly to six monthly out-patient procedure.

People Likely to be In Touch

In Hospital General physician, cardiologist, geriatrician, social worker.

At Home General practitioner, health visitor, district nurse, 'pacemaker' or cardiac out-patient clinic at the hospital.

Help Needed

Initially, the condition of heart block can cause great anxiety and distress for the patient and his family. All areas of life are affected and there is fear of imminent death. The heart is symbolic of life and any kind of heart disease, particularly the seeming cessation of the beat, is very alarming. The insertion of an artificial pacemaker comes as a great relief. The patient and family may need help to adapt, but on the whole good adjustments are made. As in most heart disease, there may be problems of changing employment or leisure activities.

Resources

Chest, Heart and Stroke Association,
Tavistock House (North),
Tavistock Square,
London WC1H 9JE.
Telephone 01 387 3012
Promotes research and wider knowledge, educational literature, cassettes.

Heart Failure/ Congestive Cardiac Failure

The Medical Condition

AGE OF ONSET Middle to old age.

CAUSE There are three main causes:

1 High blood pressure.
2 Chronic disease of the heart valves, usually years after an attack of rheumatic fever. Sometimes due to congenital heart disease – 'blue baby'.
3 An impaired blood flow from the blood vessels that supply the heart (coronary arteries).

A less common cause is chronic chest disease.

COURSE The course of events leading to heart failure is very variable, depending on the cause. High blood pressure may be detected by accident during routine examination or may go undiscovered until there is a crisis and the heart fails.

Coronary artery disease can happen suddenly when the artery becomes obstructed. This can lead to severe damage to the heart muscle. It is this condition for which patients are admitted urgently to hospital coronary care units and which can cause death. It is not usually curable, though the symptoms can be controlled.

Angina People with coronary heart disease may suffer angina before they develop heart failure. This is a severe crushing type of central chest pain which occurs usually after walking a certain distance or as a result of excitement. Although it lasts only a few minutes the patient looks and feels very ill. It can be quickly relieved by chewing tablets containing a very small dose of nitro-glycerine.

EFFECTS The two most obvious effects are shortness of breath, and a waterlogged swelling of the tissues, particularly in the legs (oedema). The patient finds it difficult to get about, climb stairs, etc. A state of chronic ill health may develop, with recurrent acute illnesses requiring bed rest or hospital admission.

TREATMENT Regular medication is required, usually with digitalis (Digoxin) and diuretics (which get rid of the excess body fluid through the kidneys). For younger people with valvular heart disease, surgical repair is often successful. Where there is high blood pressure, modern drugs are very effective in lowering this, though they can still bring unpleasant side effects. Depending on the extent of damage to the heart, life may have to be moderated and carefully planned to avoid undue physical and mental strain.

People Likely to be In Touch

In Hospital Cardiologist, general physician, cardiac surgeon, geriatrician, social worker, physiotherapist.

At Home General practitioner, district nurse, health visitor, domiciliary occupational therapist.

Help Needed

Heart disease may develop slowly giving patient and family time to adjust gradually. A sudden onset causes acute anxiety. Everyone is aware of the threat to survival and may overreact. It is important to achieve a balance between living as normal and full a life as possible and keeping within reasonable limits to preserve health. This may mean major adjustments in work and family, sexual and leisure activities. Both counselling and practical help will be needed.

CHECK LIST DHSS Benefits – Mobility Allowance, Invalidity Allowance. Aids and Adaptations – refer to domiciliary occupational therapist. Housing. Employment – Disablement Resettlement Officer. Home Help. Meals on Wheels. Day Care. Holidays. Voluntary help.

Resources

Chest, Heart and Stroke Association,
Tavistock House (North),
Tavistock Square,
London WC1H 9JE.
Telephone 01 387 3012
Helps and advises. Promotes research and wider knowledge, educational literature, cassettes.

Hodgkin's Disease

The Medical Condition

AGE OF ONSET Adults. More men than women, most common in middle age.

CAUSE This is the commonest of a variety of cancerous conditions which affect the cells of the glandular system. There is a link between these cancers and some forms of leukaemia.

COURSE Hodgkin's disease begins insidiously and painlessly, progressing to generalized illness. There is a high chance of recovery, though some forms (lymphoma) do not respond so well to treatment.

EFFECTS The first symptom is usually a lump in the neck. Later other lumps may appear in the groin, armpit, or abdomen. Then follow general symptoms such as weight loss, anaemia, debility, and fluctuating fever. There may be deep seated pain.

TREATMENT Drugs and radiotherapy (deep X-ray) can halt the spread of the disease. It is possible to be more optimistic about the outcome than in most other cancers, and at least some measure of remission can usually be achieved.

People Likely to be In Touch

In Hospital Radiotherapist, general physician, staff of radiotherapy unit, social worker.

At Home General practitioner, district nurse, health visitor, radiotherapy clinic.

Help Needed

See entry on Cancer. The same anxieties may be present as with other forms of cancer. However, the recent improvement in treatment gives much scope for reassurance to patient and family. Liaise with hospital unit and primary care team to give support during the illness and rehabilitation.

CHECK LIST DHSS Benefits. Home Help. Disablement Resettlement Officer – change of employment. Holidays.

Resources

National Society for Cancer Relief (see page 27).

Huntington's Chorea

The Medical Condition

AGE OF ONSET Usually becomes apparent between thirty-five and fifty years of age.

CAUSE Unknown. Hereditary disease transmitted by father or mother.

COURSE The course varies. There can be a rapid advance to disability and dementia or patient can be relatively unaffected through life. Not likely to reach old age.

EFFECTS Mild onset, unsteady walk, memory or mood changes. Increased fidgety movements of limbs during waking hours and slurred speech. These symptoms are accompanied by progressive mental failure.

TREATMENT Drugs to control involuntary movements and mental symptoms. In advanced stages patients are usually admitted to psychiatric hospital. Genetic counselling for families.

People Likely to be In Touch

In Hospital General physician, neurologist and/or psychiatrist, social worker, occupational therapist.

At Home General practitioner, district nurse, psychiatric hospital day unit, young disabled unit, domiciliary occupational therapist.

Help Needed

In the early stages, Huntington's chorea should be regarded in the same way as any disabling condition. Patients should not be labelled mentally ill although the psychiatrist needs to be alerted because of the possible long-term effects. Constant support and help is needed by the family throughout the deterioration of the patient. Liaison with other professionals to assess need and identify key worker. Children in family may need help, special problems arise because of hereditary factor. Periodic admissions to hospital may be arranged in order to share the care with the family.

CHECK LIST DHSS Benefits, e.g. Attendance Allowance, Invalid Care Allowance. Day Care/Day Hospital. Aids – refer to occupational therapist. Permanent residential care. Home Help. Holidays. Voluntary help.

Resources

Association to Combat Huntington's Chorea,
Lyndhurst,
Lower Hampton Road,
Sunbury-on-Thames,
Middlesex TW16 5PR.
Telephone 01 979 5055
Provides help of all kinds. Booklets of information for families and doctors.

Also run Holiday/Short Stay Home.

Combat Holiday Home,
Theydon Road,
Epping,
Essex CM16 4DX.
Telephone 0378 77588
Offers short stay for patient or patient and spouse. Aids and equipment are available to try and counselling is offered.

Hypertension

(High Blood Pressure)

The Medical Condition

AGE OF ONSET Middle life. Men are more commonly and more severely affected.

CAUSE Many factors. There may be an inherited tendency, aggravated by excess weight, smoking, stress, excess of salt or dairy products in diet, previous kidney disease.

COURSE High blood pressure is often accidentally discovered during a routine medical examination. Sometimes there are early signs such as headaches or giddiness. The course after this will depend on medication and the patient's life style.

EFFECTS The rise in pressure inside the blood vessels may produce no direct symptoms, but the damage to the arteries supplying different organs may lead to any of the following:
retinal (eye) changes and poor vision (see page 22)
stroke (see page 122)
arteriosclerotic dementia (see page 13)
heart failure (see page 65)
angina (see page 65)
kidney (renal) failure (see page 74)
People with this condition are often obsessively anxious and take on a heavy load of life's commitments. They may see their condition as an extra burden or a welcome excuse to slow down.

TREATMENT Constant treatment by drugs in an attempt to keep the blood pressure at a lower level. Regular medical checks are necessary, as is advice about diet and a change to a more moderate and healthy way of life. A *mild* rise in blood pressure in middle age may need no treatment.

People Likely to be In Touch

In Hospital General physician, geriatrician, dietician, social worker.

At Home General practitioner, district nurse.

Help Needed

'Blood pressure' is regarded with respect by most people. It is invisible and can generate alarm and misunderstanding. It can be a warning of a more serious illness. People may respond to it by (a) ignoring it and stopping medication and (b) using it as a threat to manipulate other people or get out of unpleasant situations, and therefore it can be part of personal or family problems presented to the worker. Social workers should liaise with the general practitioner where the extent of the medical problem is uncertain.

CHECK LIST DHSS Benefits. Disablement Resettlement Officer – change of employment. Holidays.

Hypothermia

The Medical Condition

AGE OF ONSET Any age. Babies and old people are the most vulnerable.

CAUSE The body has regulating mechanisms that will not allow the temperature to rise or fall beyond a certain limited range. Babies and very old people have relatively poor control of these mechanisms, especially in a cold environment. There is a fall in body temperature from the normal 98.4°F to 90°F or even 80°F.

COURSE As the body cools, normal shivering tends to disappear and the patient may not complain of the cold. A temperature below 95°F is significant. Anything below 90°F is dangerous. Survival is unlikely below 85°F.

EFFECTS Old people with a lowered temperature tend to become slightly confused and slow moving. They may not be aware of their cold environment and will not therefore take appropriate action, such as putting on warmer clothes or lighting a fire. Hands and feet may naturally be cold, but if the skin on the abdomen feels cold to the touch, this is a danger signal. Small babies, who have a large skin surface in relation to their body weight, lose heat easily and are very susceptible to cold.

TREATMENT Hypothermia is usually only discovered in a crisis. The elderly patient at home is normally admitted promptly to hospital and slowly warmed up. It should be noted that this condition can occur in hospital or residential home if heating is inadequate and old people immobile for long periods. The condition is liable to recur. Prevention is better than cure, and a crisis can be averted by the provision of adequate heating, warm clothing, and a proper diet. The morning living room temperature should be at least 65°F. (18.3°C.) (A room thermometer is useful.) Bedrooms are generally colder and warm bedclothes, an electric blanket, and background heating during the night should be available.

People Likely to be In Touch

In Hospital General physician, geriatrician, paediatrician, social worker, occupational therapist.

At Home General practitioner, health visitor, domiciliary occupational therapist, day hospital/centre.

These patients are usually referred in a crisis. Hypothermia may be the first warning of problems of isolation, depression, poverty, or the inability to manage alone. A full assessment must be made, and anything from practical and supportive services at home to residential care may be needed. Old people are often afraid of spending money on heating and food. They can be unaware of the extra benefits to which they are entitled. They may be unable to cope with some forms of heating, or need encouragement to use an electric blanket.

CHECK LIST DHSS Benefits and all extra allowances for heating, clothing, food. Home Help. Domiciliary occupational therapist for aids to daily living. Meals on Wheels. Good Neighbour Schemes and Volunteers to visit regularly. Day Care. Lunch Clubs. Periodic/permanent residential care.

Resources

1 Community Physicians and Health Visitors – Health Authority Community Sector.
2 Emergency heating equipment or fuel is available from Social Services Departments.
3 Weekly extra heating allowance can be claimed from DHSS Supplementary Benefits Commission and grants towards heating appliances may be allowed.
4 Electricity and Gas Boards can advise and help with suitable appliances, tariff, and easy payment schemes.
5 Local charities and voluntary organizations such as Age Concern may be able to help with small heating allowances or one-off grants.
6 British Red Cross Society (local branch).
7 Good Neighbour Schemes.
8 See Dr Muir Gray's book *Take Care of your Elderly Relative*. Chapter 8.

Kidney Failure (Chronic)

The Medical Condition

AGE OF ONSET Any age.

CAUSE Chronic kidney disease, which until recent years proved fatal. Often treated now by renal dialysis and/or transplantation of kidneys.

COURSE May be sudden and complete kidney failure or a slow deterioration over months, and even years. The course varies according to the suitability of the patient for dialysis or transplantation.

EFFECTS This disease is serious and distressing and disrupts family life, especially during the machine dialysis stage, which for some may last for years. Initially patients feel ill on dialysis. They improve, but then have to face being dependent on a dialysis machine two or three times a week unless they can have a successful transplant. Suicidal depression is common and some may refuse treatment. Once this stage is past, people adjust in varying degrees to this dependency. There is heavy reliance on the hospital team, and dialysis at home imposes extra stresses on patient and family, which are sometimes disruptive.

TREATMENT *Dialysis* means being regularly linked to a machine which substitutes the function of the kidneys in eliminating waste products from the blood stream. Patients start treatment in hospital and they and their partner (spouse, parent, friend) are taught to use the machine in preparation for dialysing at home. They must usually dialyse three times a week, often at night, and for periods up to six hours. They cannot normally be left unattended while on the machine.

Transplant Surgery People can live normally with one kidney, so healthy people can donate a kidney if there is a close biological match with the patient. Many things can go wrong after surgery, but if all goes well, people can lead normal lives. They will however need special drugs for years and some will need further transplants.

People Likely to be In Touch

In Hospital The whole team in the Renal Unit, i.e. doctor, nurse, social worker, technician, psychiatrist, administrator. Patient is likely to remain in constant touch with this team, rather than with primary care team at home.

At Home General practitioner, district nurse, social worker (especially if long distance from Renal Unit). Structural alterations for installation of kidney machine are dealt with by hospital and local authority, with special central monies – not Social Services Department.

Help Needed

Adjustment to dialysis depends a great deal on previous family strengths. Although the patient may be in touch with the hospital team, other family members may need counselling and support. Particular strain is placed on marital relationships and sexual counselling may be necessary. Children with kidney diseases are very often over-protected, become self-centred, and suffer from the effects of disrupted education and abnormal social development. Dialysis for children has special complications. Workers may be asked to counsel and support families who live a long distance from Unit and become involved in other family problems, e.g. children before courts, or elderly parents, etc. In all cases it is essential to liaise closely with Renal Unit social worker.

CHECK LIST DHSS Benefits – Attendance Allowance. Special Diet Allowance.

Resources

British Kidney Patients Association,
Bordon,
Hampshire.
Telephone Bordon (042 03) 2022
Gives advice and help to sufferers, fund raising, encourages donation of kidneys. Holiday units available with machine installed.

Local group for support, social events and advice. See BASW Publication *Social Workers Caring for Patients with Chronic Renal Failure.*

Leukaemia (Acute)

The Medical Condition

AGE OF ONSET Usually affects children and young adults.

CAUSE It is a malignant disease due to overgrowth of white cells in the bone marrow, increasing rapidly, and usually affecting the whole bloodstream. The malignant white cells displace the normal ones so that the patient becomes anaemic, vulnerable to infection, and liable to bleed.

COURSE The disease begins insidiously and may have been present for some time before it is noticed. (It may be picked up at a routine blood test.) The course of the disease is dependent on the patient's response to treatment and his vulnerability to infection. A proportion of children reach a 'five year cure', but treatment is hazardous and the sudden death of a patient is always possible. Adults are often more difficult to treat and there is much less chance of recovery.

EFFECTS The first symptoms may follow an infection which clears up too slowly, or a bleeding episode, for instance after a dental extraction. Patients feel ill, debilitated, and lethargic.

TREATMENT This entails hospitalization, and normally a great deal of counselling is done by medical and nursing staff at ward level. Drug treatment may result in the child looking unpleasantly plump and 'bonny'. The patient is very liable to infection and therefore normal schooling is impossible, and even parents may be excluded from being with the child at times. Sudden relapses frequently occur, needing emergency measures such as blood transfusions.

People Likely to be In Touch

In Hospital Paediatrician, haematologist, general physician, social worker for paediatric unit, children's ward staff, children's day unit. Parents may be involved in a self help group.

At Home General practitioner, health visitor.

Help Needed

Counselling of patient and parents will more than likely be covered by hospital staff. There is intense anxiety and uncertainty surrounding this illness and other siblings may need to be cared for in parents' absence (hospital attendance and visiting) and counselled in their own right. In the event of death, bereavement work will need to continue after the link with hospital is broken. Liaise closely with hospital staff and the primary health care team.

CHECK LIST DHSS Benefits. Home Help. Outings and holidays for siblings. Fares for visiting hospital – DHSS or Charity.

Resources

Leukaemia Society,
Hon. Sec. Mr David Harding,
186 Torbay Road,
Rayners Lane,
Harrow,
Middlesex HA2 9QL.
Telephone 01 868 4107
Local branches throughout the country for help, support, and information.

National Society for Cancer Relief,
Michael Sobell House,
30 Dorset Square,
London NW1 6QL.
Telephone 01 402 8125
Will give money for specific purposes or weekly grants for people at home. Usually make rapid response to requests. They also help to fund a network of terminal care units in conjunction with the NHS.

Leukaemia (Chronic)

The Medical Condition

AGE OF ONSET Late middle age and onwards.

CAUSE An overgrowth of white cells in the bone marrow, which displace the normal ones so that the patient becomes anaemic.

COURSE This is a much less serious condition than acute leukaemia. It is often discovered by chance at a routine physical examination. It may last for years in a benign state and life expectancy is not necessarily affected. A few cases may eventually become acute. (See page 76 for Acute Leukaemia.)

EFFECTS The patient may only show mild anaemia, and vague abdominal discomfort because of the enlargement of the spleen.

TREATMENT Some patients may have this disease for years without requiring any treatment at all. Others will need drugs to maintain health, or more rarely, blood transfusion. Regular hospital out-patient check ups are necessary.

People Likely to be In Touch

In Hospital Haematologist, general physician, social worker.
At Home General practitioner.

Help Needed

Leukaemia is usually considered to be a frightening and life-threatening disease, and it may be important to help a patient and his family to understand the benign nature of chronic leukaemia, and to plan optimistically for the future. It will be necessary to work closely with the general practitioner. The disease affects older people, and may coincide with problems of retirement, loss of spouse, and change of accommodation etc. Special counselling and support may be necessary.

CHECK LIST DHSS Benefits. Home Help.

Leukaemia Society,
Hon. Sec. Mr David Harding,
186 Torbay Road,
Rayners Lane,
Harrow,
Middlesex HA2 9QL.
Telephone 01 868 4107
Local branches throughout the country for help, support, and information.

Ménière's Disease

The Medical Condition

AGE OF ONSET Usually over fifty, more common in women.

CAUSE The precise cause is unknown. It is a chronic progressive condition of the inner ear which is concerned with balance as well as hearing.

COURSE Attacks can occur in clusters but there may be long intervals when the patient is symptom free. In severe cases there is a gradual increasing deafness in the affected ear, and it is possible that both ears may be damaged, leading ultimately to complete deafness.

EFFECTS The patient is seized by an acute attack of severe giddiness. There is usually a buzzing noise in the ears (tinnitus) and she often falls to the ground. She may have severe nausea and vomiting and have to stay in bed. She will feel extremely frightened of moving. The acute attack lasts between fifteen minutes and an hour, but it may take much longer for the patient to recover completely.

TREATMENT There is no cure for this condition. Symptoms can be treated by drugs, and sometimes surgical treatment is helpful.

People Likely to be In Touch

In Hospital Ear Nose and Throat Surgeon or clinic team, hearing aid clinic, hearing therapist.

At Home General practitioner, health visitor, ENT hospital out-patient clinic, specialist social worker for the deaf.

Help Needed

By the time this condition becomes disabling it is likely that the patient will be elderly. The attacks are very alarming, and there may be hidden fears and anxiety associated with them. The increasing deafness brings special problems and patients may require help in combating isolation and overcoming communication problems.

Resources

Voluntary Organizations for the Deaf (see Deafness, page 44).

Migraine

The Medical Condition

AGE OF ONSET Can date from early childhood, but most commonly appears about the age of puberty.

CAUSE A paroxysmal nervous disturbance leading to intense headache which can be precipitated by various trigger factors, e.g. certain foods or drink, social pressures, etc. Migraine sufferers are commonly of a certain personality type, energetic, intelligent, with a strong obsessional streak.

COURSE Migraine is a common form of recurrent headache. These headaches usually occur in clusters, and there may be long clear periods, possibly months, in between. In women, migraine often ceases at the menopause, and in either sex it rarely persists into old age. The sexes are equally affected, and a family history is common.

EFFECTS Migraine sufferers are usually otherwise healthy. The attack may start on waking in the morning with giddiness, visual disturbance and nausea. Sometimes there are premonitory signs, e.g. a halo aura around lights. This is followed by a severe pounding headache, often accompanied by vomiting. Sufferers may be completely prostrated for several hours and have to lie down in a darkened room. They may be unable to cope with anything until the following morning, when they feel shaken by the episode, but otherwise well. In childhood, the nausea, vomiting, and prostration may be more pronounced than the headache which can confuse the diagnosis.

TREATMENT The tendency cannot be cured, but various medications can be given to reduce the frequency of attacks and mitigate their severity. Early recognition of the first signs of an attack is important. Sometimes it may be possible to ward off an attack altogether by prompt treatment. Special clinics for migraine have been set up throughout the country, and sufferers should attend these in order to get specialist care.

People Likely to be In Touch

In Hospital Physician at migraine clinic (if available).
At Home General practitioner.

Help Needed

Many people suffer from migraine during the most productive years of their lives, and it can have serious effects on their work and happiness. It may be possible to help them to eliminate precipitating stress factors if these can be identified. Temporary help with children may be needed for certain patients, such as one parent families. It is essential that the child's school should understand a child's susceptibility to migraine and be able to cope with an attack.

CHECK LIST Family Aide. Daily Minder. Volunteer – for parents with migraine who need help with young children.

Resources

British Migraine Association,
Evergreen,
Ottermead Lane,
Ottershaw,
Chertsey, Surrey CT16 0HJ.
Offers hope, help, and the latest research news.

Migraine Trust,
45 Great Ormond Street,
London WC1.
Telephone 01 741 7833
Good literature, advice, and list of clinics can be obtained.

Mongolism

(Down's Syndrome)

The Medical Condition

AGE OF ONSET Birth.

CAUSE Congenital abnormality due to a chromosome defect. Often found in children born to elderly mothers.

COURSE These children in the past seldom survived beyond adolescence, but now many live well into adult life. Some are born with other abnormalities such as defective heart valves and are more likely to die in childhood or teens.

EFFECTS These vary according to the degree of handicap. The child has from infancy a short, broad face, and slanting eyelids, sometimes without eyelashes, and often a protruding tongue. His hands are short fingered, broad and clumsy. His intelligence is low and learning ability limited, although some will achieve a much higher level. He may have some minor physical handicap as well, and more than other children be susceptible to infections. The mongol child is usually cheerful, amiable, and very charming.

TREATMENT There is no cure for this condition. Infections or other complications are treated in the usual way. Genetic counselling and screening is now available to pregnant women over the age of thirty-five years.

People Likely to be In Touch

In Hospital Paediatrician, special care baby unit, social worker, paediatric assessment centre, day unit at subnormality hospital.

At Home General practitioner, health visitor, special playgroup or nursery, special school (Education Department), school counsellor, school medical officer (Health Department), adult training centre, special clubs for mentally handicapped, local voluntary parents group.

Help Needed

The referral may come from the hospital social worker after the birth of a mongol child. It is important in any case to liaise with the hospital team. Mothers may have great difficulty in coming to terms with the birth and some may reject the baby initially.

There will almost certainly be need for support from hospital and community social workers, general practitioner and health visitor from an early stage. Parents need information about available help and services from the start. Reception into care may be necessary, short or long term. In the beginning, mongol children are much like normal babies. It is later, in terms of milestones, that parents realize the extent of handicap. Social work may only be required intermittently, but it is important that parents know where to obtain help at any time from a 'named' person. There is a need for forward planning e.g. consideration of special or residential school, hostel etc. Parents can easily become over-protective and anxious and other siblings may suffer. In adulthood there may be special problems, e.g. where elderly parents are no longer able to cope. A great deal of social work help may be required to enable a transfer to alternative care.

CHECK LIST DHSS Benefits – Attendance Allowance. Special School Holidays. Periodic/permanent residential care (Hostel, Hospital). Playgroups. Voluntary Help Groups, Clubs, etc. Toy Libraries.

Resources

Down's Children's Association,
Quinborne Community Centre,
Ridgacre Road,
Quinton,
Birmingham B32 2TW.
Telephone 021 427 1374
Gives advice on the developmental management of mongol children and the promotion of research into care and education.

National Society for Mentally Handicapped Children and Adults (MENCAP),
117-123 Golden Lane,
London EC1Y 0RT.
Telephone 01 253 9433
Local branches. Regional Offices. Gateway Clubs for Seniors and Juniors. Residential homes. Welfare visitors.

Motor Neurone Disease

The Medical Condition

AGE OF ONSET Usually between thirty and fifty years of age. Predominantly males.

CAUSE Unknown.

COURSE Variable. Usually a gradual onset of symptoms. Deterioration and disablement occurs over a period of months or years, leading to death. (Average expectation of life is two to three years.)

EFFECTS Weakness and wasting of the muscles, most commonly the hands, shoulder and neck. The patient becomes totally dependent and speech, swallowing, and breathing can become difficult, and finally impossible.

TREATMENT No curative treatment is known. Some drugs may alleviate symptoms. Physiotherapy and good nursing care can help and comfort.

People Likely to be In Touch

In Hospital Neurologist, general physician, social worker, occupational therapist, physiotherapist.

At Home General practitioner, district nurse, Cottage Hospital, Young Disabled Unit, Terminal Care Unit.

Help Needed

Because of the relatively short duration and distressing nature of this condition, there is a need for maximum practical and psychological help to patient and family. Liaise with hospital staff, primary health care team, and occupational therapist. Short term admissions may be necessary and terminal care provided. Bereavement counselling may be necessary.

CHECK LIST DHSS Benefits, e.g. Attendance Allowance, Mobility Allowance, Invalid Care Allowance. Aids and Adaptations – refer to occupational therapist. Home Help. Meals on Wheels. Day Care. Voluntary help.

Resources

General Organizations for the Disabled (see page 133).
Local voluntary groups or charities may assist families.

86 Motor Neurone Disease Association,
Secretary Mrs E. Ann Grelton,
7 Lorimer Avenue,
Gedling,
Nottingham,
or Miss Hilary Major,
209 Pickhurst Lane,
West Wickham,
Kent BR4 0HH
Telephone (evenings only) 01 462 7348

Multiple Sclerosis

(Also known as disseminated sclerosis)

The Medical Condition

AGE OF ONSET Most frequently develops in young adults and rarely after age fifty-five.

CAUSE Unknown.

COURSE Usually gradual onset, often small warning signs such as double vision, pins and needles in limbs, long before diagnosis can be made. The course of the disease is variable, some people progressing rapidly to complete disability while others may have only mild relapses and long remissions throughout life, with minimum permanent effects. Death usually occurs before old age.

EFFECTS The disease affects the central nervous system and is characterized by relapses and remissions. It can therefore interfere with the normal function of most parts of the body. Ordinary daily living can be restricted by excessive feelings of fatigue. Symptoms include paralysis of limbs, muscle tremor and spasm, slurred speech, incontinence, and affected eyesight. Some patients are confined to wheelchair living and are prone to chest and urinary infections.

TREATMENT No curative treatment has been found. Cortisone is given during acute episodes to reduce symptoms. Physiotherapy is found to be beneficial by the patient. Energy needs to be conserved and extremes of heat and cold avoided. Because no effective medical treatment can be offered people very often try fringe remedies such as diet and exercise routines, faith healers, etc.

People Likely to be In Touch

In Hospital Neurologist, general physician, specialist in rehabilitation, social workers, occupational therapist, physiotherapist.

At Home General practitioner, health visitor, district nurse, domiciliary occupational therapist, Multiple Sclerosis Society, Volunteers, Day Centre/Hospital, Out-patient physiotherapy, neurology clinic.

Help Needed

A thorough assessment of present position with patient, family, and other professionals involved. The family are facing a long term problem with recurring crises, and therefore with changing needs. Because of the deteriorating process of the disease, frequent re-assessment is necessary by all professionals involved. Early and constant support to the family/carer is important and may avoid the breakdown of marriage/relationships, which so often happens during the progress of this illness. Hospitals and Social Service Departments should share the care with the family by offering programmed admissions. Sexual counselling may be necessary.

CHECK LIST DHSS Benefits, e.g. Attendance and Mobility Allowances. Disabled Housewives Allowance. Invalid Care Allowance. Motability. Day Care. Aids and Adaptations – refer to occupational therapist. Housing. Employment – Disablement Resettlement Officer. Home Help. Meals on Wheels. Intermittent/permanent residential care. Holidays. Voluntary help.

Resources

Multiple Sclerosis Society of Great Britain and Northern Ireland,
286 Munster Road,
Fulham,
London SW6 6AP.
Telephone 01 381 4022/5
Promotes research. Provides, through local branches, advice, social activities, holidays, financial aid, and visiting.

CRACK MS self help groups aim to meet the welfare and social needs of young people with multiple sclerosis.

ARMS,
71 Grays Inn Road,
London WC1X 8TR.
24 Hour Counselling Service. Telephone 01 568 2255.

Muscular Dystrophy

(Duchenne Type)

The Medical Condition

AGE OF ONSET Birth.

CAUSE Unknown. Hereditary disease, predominantly males. Passed on by unaffected females.

COURSE Parents first notice that child walks badly and has difficulty in picking himself up and climbing stairs. The muscles become weak and there is a gradual deterioration leading eventually to death. Very few reach adult life.

EFFECTS Large children with seemingly overdeveloped muscles. Often become fat, heavy, and wheelchair bound, and therefore difficult to manage. Very prone to chest infection. There is no mental abnormality.

TREATMENT No curative treatment is known. Family need genetic counselling, which will be arranged by doctor.

People Likely to be In Touch

In Hospital Paediatrician, neurologist, and social worker.

At Home General practitioner, health visitor, district nurse, domiciliary occupational therapist, Education department, school, home teacher.

Help Needed

Assess need with child and family, and primary health care team. There are sometimes two children affected in one family and parents will need support through the dying, and the loss of both of them. Other siblings may need help in their own right. Careful liaison with other workers involved for bereavement counselling, for example the home teacher may be the person most closely involved.

CHECK LIST DHSS Benefits – Attendance Allowance. Aids and Adaptations – refer to occupational therapist. Home Help to relieve mother. Periodic/permanent residential care. Holidays. Leisure activities for disabled child.

Muscular Dystrophy Group of Great Britain,
Nattrass House,
35 Macaulay Road,
London SW4 0QP.
Telephone 01 720 8055
Primarily a medical research charity, but will help and advise sufferers. Handbook and literature. Local branch in most areas.

See Helpful Organizations for Children (page 136).

Myasthenia Gravis

The Medical Condition

AGE OF ONSET Adult life, usually twenty to thirty, predominantly women.

CAUSE Unknown.

COURSE This is an illness characterized by extreme muscle fatigue, beginning slowly, with a gradual build up of symptoms. Its course is extremely variable. In some cases symptoms are very severe, and there are breathing difficulties from which complications may arise leading to death. In others the illness only affects small groups of muscles and there may be long periods of remission.

EFFECTS

The patient may first notice a variety of symptoms such as drooping eyelids, double vision, difficulty in swallowing, and the voice may become progressively weak and husky. The weakness improves with rest. Patients feel well early in the morning, but symptoms appear during the day. Arm muscles may be involved and routine tasks such as doing the hair may become very difficult. Chewing can become virtually impossible towards evening and the neck muscles are unable to support the head. The whole body can be affected and breathing and swallowing become hazardous.

TREATMENT By drugs and sometimes surgical removal of the thymus gland. Patients very often need admission to hospital because of breathing difficulties.

People Likely to be In Touch

In Hospital Neurologist, occupational therapist, respiration unit staff, social worker for neurology unit.

At Home General practitioner, health visitor, domiciliary occupational therapist.

Help Needed

Need to work closely with hospital social worker. Family help may be needed, for example if mother is admitted to hospital possibly for a long period. Myasthenia is not a well-known illness and sufferers benefit particularly from contact with the voluntary society, where their condition is well understood.

The symptoms, if severe, are very unsightly for family and patient. There can be effects on sexual and family relationships and work.

CHECK LIST DHSS Benefits – Mobility Allowance, Disabled Housewives Allowance. Aids – refer to occupational therapist. Home Help. Meals on Wheels.

Resources

Myasthenia Gravis Council of Muscular Dystrophy Group of Great Britain,
Nattrass House,
35 Macaulay Road,
London SW4 0QP.
Telephone 01 720 8055
There is a network of contacts throughout the British Isles. This is a self help patients group and the Co-ordinator is:
Mrs Marjorie Rivett,
38 Selwood Road,
Brentwood, Essex.
Telephone 0277 218082
Regular bulletins are issued and Mrs Rivett holds the mailing list and register of patients.

Paget's Disease

The Medical Condition

AGE OF ONSET Middle to old age.

CAUSE Abnormal changes in the bone.

COURSE Mild Paget's disease can be free of symptoms and undetected. The most severe examples are chronically painful and disabling. The change in appearance is so gradual that it is usually taken as part of the ageing process.

EFFECTS The disease can affect the legs, pelvis, spine, and skull. In the affected area the bone tends to swell, soften, and become more liable to fracture. The bones of the legs and spine may bend. If the forehead is affected this produces a bulging appearance. There may be progressive deafness. Bone pain can be severe and the disabling effects are similar to chronic arthritis.

TREATMENT There is no curative treatment, but pain can be controlled by hormone injections. Keeping active and mobile is important and can be encouraged by physiotherapy.

People Likely to be In Touch

In Hospital Physician, rheumatologist, geriatrician, physiotherapist, occupational therapist, social worker, day hospital.

At Home General practitioner, health visitor, domiciliary occupational therapist, day centre/hospital

Help Needed

Paget's disease brings extra complications to the already existing problems of elderly people. There is a higher risk than usual of breaking a bone and therefore special aids and adaptations around the home may be needed. People may need help with housework, shopping, and transport, and in advanced severe cases periodic or permanent residential care may be necessary.

CHECK LIST DHSS Benefits – Attendance Allowance, Special Heating Allowance. Aids and Adaptations – refer to domiciliary occupational therapist. Home Help. Voluntary Services. Special Housing. Holidays. Periodic/permanent residential care.

National Association for the Relief of Paget's Disease,
Secretary, Mrs A. Stansfield,
413 Middleton Road,
Middleton,
Manchester M24 4QZ.
Promotes research and offers mutual support to patients. General organizations for the elderly, e.g. Age Concern.

Parkinson's Disease

The Medical Condition

AGE OF ONSET Middle age onwards. More men than women.

CAUSE Unknown.

COURSE Insidious onset of symptoms, which are progressively disabling. Now usually well controlled by drugs.

EFFECTS The disease is characterized by shaking, muscle weakness and rigidity, stooping posture, shuffling walk. The face may become mask-like and immobile. Because of recent developments in drugs, it is unusual to see full blown cases of Parkinson's disease today.

TREATMENT There is no known cure, but drugs such as L-Dopa, Amantadine, and Artane, are now very effective. Patients may need hospital admission to establish dosage. Physiotherapy can be very useful.

People Likely to be In Touch

In Hospital Physician, neurologist, geriatrician, physiotherapist, occupational therapist, social worker.

At Home General practitioner, health visitor, domiciliary occupational therapist, day care/hospital.

Help Needed

Although drug treatment is now much more effective, some patients will still be substantially disabled by tremor, weakness, and speech difficulty. In these cases, employment and family relationships will be affected and at times residential care may be necessary. Parkinsonism is essentially a disease of the decline of life and will therefore be part of work with frail elderly.

CHECK LIST DHSS Benefits, e.g. Attendance Allowance, Invalid Care Allowance, Extra Heating Allowance. Aids and Adaptations – refer to occupational therapist. Housing. Home Help. Meals on Wheels. Day Care. Periodic or permanent residential care.

Parkinson's Disease Society of the UK Ltd,
81 Queens Road,
London SW19 8NR.
Telephone 01 946 2500
Organizes local groups, offers support to patients and families. Literature and information available.

See General Organizations for the Disabled (page 133).
Voluntary Organizations for the Elderly.

Peptic Ulcer

(Gastric, Duodenal Ulcer)

The Medical Condition

AGE OF ONSET Early adulthood onwards. More common in males than females.

CAUSE The initiating cause is unknown but the ulcer is aggravated by the acid and digestive juices from the stomach, which in turn can be affected by stress, anxiety, and smoking.

COURSE The ulcer develops in the stomach or more commonly in the first part of the intestine (duodenum) into which the food passes from the stomach. The condition may remain chronic, being intermittently troublesome for years. If it becomes acute, there are symptoms of indigestion and abdominal pain. The ulcer may suddenly bleed profusely and blood is vomited up or passed through the bowel. There may be perforation of the stomach wall and the contents of the stomach or duodenum are released into the abdominal cavity. The patient will need emergency admission for medical and surgical treatment after which recovery is normally good.

EFFECTS The common symptom is pain recurring regularly about one and a half to two hours after food. During acute attacks the pain is more intense and the condition can become life threatening. The chronic ill health sometimes associated with this condition can produce an introspective semi-invalid who can be demanding on other people.

TREATMENT Alkaline mixtures and tablets are given to neutralize the acids and other more specific medicines are nowadays very effective. Emergency surgical treatment may be needed for an acute episode. When symptoms have been difficult to control or there have been recurrent complications, more drastic surgery may be required to cut down the amount of acid produced in the stomach or to remove the damaged area. Patients frequently develop food fads but it is questionable whether special diets are beneficial except during the first few weeks of treatment.

People Likely to be In Touch

In Hospital Physician, surgeon, social worker, dietician.
At Home General practitioner, district nurse.

Help Needed

This condition may be a component of social problems which are causing stress and anxiety. If the social worker can help to alleviate these problems, e.g. financial, housing, marital, this may contribute to the success of the treatment. Work should be in conjunction with the general practitioner.

CHECK LIST DHSS Benefits – Family Income Supplement. Housing. Financial help from charities. Holidays. Convalescence.

Resources

Convalescent Homes – National Health Service arrange direct from hospital. See Union Convalescent Homes. Charities Digest – for financial help.

Perthes' Disease of the Hip

The Medical Condition

AGE OF ONSET Childhood, five to ten years. Boys affected more than girls.

CAUSE Unknown. A degenerative condition of the head of the femur (long bone of the leg).

COURSE If diagnosis is made as soon as symptoms appear, with treatment the child may return to full activity. There is a risk of osteoarthritis in later life.

EFFECTS The hip bone is temporarily softened and there is risk of deformity if the child continues normal activities. The bone eventually returns to normal consistency. The child has pain in the groin or thigh, muscle spasm, and walks with a limp.

TREATMENT By admission to hospital for immobilization and surgery to correct the position of the bones. The child will then spend some time at home in plaster before readmission to hospital for removal of the plaster and rehabilitation.

People Likely to be In Touch

In Hospital Orthopaedic surgeon, paediatrician, occupational therapist, social worker, hospital teacher.

At Home General practitioner, health visitor, district nurse, home teacher, domiciliary occupational therapist.

Help Needed

Periods spent in hospital can disrupt the development of the child and education. Normal family life is affected. Parents may live long distances from hospital and find visiting and the care of other children difficult. Sometimes they may need to stay in the hospital or nearby. Workers should liaise closely with the hospital and primary health care team in offering help.

CHECK LIST DHSS Benefits – fares for visiting hospital. Temporary foster home. Family aide. Daily minder. Voluntary help. Home Help.

Perthes' Disease Group,
Mrs. R. Sawyer,
61 Wickfield Road,
Hackenthorpe,
Sheffield.

See Helpful Organizations for Children (page 136) for visiting and other expenses.

Pneumoconiosis

Asbestosis caused by Asbestos Dust
Byssinosis caused by Cotton Dust
Silicosis caused by Stone Dust
Miner's Lung caused by Coal Dust

The Medical Condition

AGE OF ONSET During working life.

CAUSE Inhalation, usually at work, of dust containing silica or certain types of fibre. Some people are far more susceptible than others.

COURSE The dust, when breathed in over a long period of time, may set up a chronic inflammation which can lead to fibrous scarring throughout the lungs. The condition is increasingly disabling and incurable.

EFFECTS The patient suffers from chronic ill health and increasing shortness of breath. The lungs become prone to infections, including tuberculosis, and in some conditions, i.e. asbestosis, lung cancer can develop.

TREATMENT Palliative only, although if infections occur, antibiotics can be used. Patients may attend the local chest clinic in hospital or an industrial rehabilitation centre. Physiotherapy can increase breathing capacity. Warm and dry living conditions are essential, and above all removal from the damaging dust.

People Likely to be In Touch

In Hospital Chest physician, general physician, physiotherapist, health visitor (chest clinic), social worker, occupational therapist.

At Home General practitioner, health visitor, domiciliary occupational therapist, industrial rehabilitation centre staff, welfare officer or personnel department at work. Disablement Resettlement Officer.

Help Needed

Dust diseases have been the subject of much research and legislation. These diseases carry a weight of blame against society and industrial development. Attitudes to them are therefore different from other illnesses. Patients can be heavily compensated financially, and special schemes are sometimes set up for holidays or residential care. Families may bear much resentment as patients become more disabled and some patients may use their condition to ensure more material and emotional help than might normally be justified. It is the wage earner of the family who is usually affected and may have to stop work. This may cause financial and family problems such as role reversal in marriage, loss of self image, and depression. Families will need practical help to ensure that housing and social conditions are as good as possible, and counselling to help adapt to different life patterns and relationships. The patient may need a change of occupation and possibly retraining, or some diversion if he is not capable of work.

CHECK LIST Special DHSS Allowances (Industrial). Mobility Allowance. Extra Heating Allowance. Rehousing. Aids and Adaptations – refer to occupational therapist. Disablement Resettlement Officer for retraining and redeployment. Periodic/permanent residential care. Holidays.

Resources

Chest, Heart and Stroke Association,
Tavistock House (North),
Tavistock Square,
London WC1H 9JE.
Telephone 01 387 3012
Promotes research and wider knowledge, educational literature, cassettes.

Employers and Union Welfare Funds and Convalescent Homes.

Pre-Senile Dementia

The Medical Condition

AGE OF ONSET Late forties to fifties onwards.

CAUSE The commonest form is arteriosclerotic (narrowing of the arteries) due to high blood pressure. In other types such as Alzheimer's Disease and Jakob Kreutzfeldt Disease the cause is unknown.

COURSE The patient can deteriorate over a few months to several years. In the final stages resistance to infection is reduced. The patient becomes extremely debilitated, ill, and finally dies.

EFFECTS The symptoms vary from person to person, but usually begin with loss of memory for recent events. The ability to solve problems becomes impaired, tactlessness and slovenly behaviour develop, and there is a general deterioration in all functioning. Incontinence and lack of inhibition emerge and in the final stages the family are left with an adult baby on their hands, who may not even recognize them. In the early stages the patient may feel depressed by his condition, but later is usually unaware of what is happening.

TREATMENT There is no curative treatment, but drugs are used to modify abnormal behaviour and assist sleeping. Day hospital and short term admissions are helpful in giving relatives relief.

People Likely to be In Touch

In Hospital Physician, neurologist, geriatrician, psychiatrist, psychologist, social worker, physiotherapist, occupational therapist.

At Home General practitioner, district nurse, community psychiatric nurse, domiciliary occupational therapist.

Help Needed

In the early stages of the disease, families can usually look after the patient at home. Later the symptoms may become unmanageable and admission to hospital or nursing home is necessary. Relatives and friends find the personality change and degradation of behaviour particularly hard to witness. They will need maximum help while the patient is still at home.

CHECK LIST DHSS Benefits: Attendance Allowance, Invalid Care Allowance, Disabled Housewives Allowance. Aids and adaptations. Domiciliary occupational therapist. Home Help. Meals on Wheels. Incontinent Laundry Service. Night sitting schemes. Day care in Centre or Hospital. Programmed intermittent/permanent residential care (usually in hospital). Voluntary visitors and 'sitters'.

Resources

Alzheimer's Disease Society,
Membership Co-ordinator Mrs C. Phillips,
Flat 6,
Bromley College,
London Road,
Bromley,
Kent BR1 1PE.
Telephone 01 464 2694
Promotes research and helps to set up support groups for relatives.

Elderly Invalids Fund,
10 Fleet Street,
London EC4.
Telephone 01 353 1892
Information on accommodation, finance, care, holidays. May provide financial help towards nursing home fees.

Psoriasis

The Medical Condition

AGE OF ONSET Usually in early adulthood.

CAUSE An abnormality in skin cell formation. The disease often runs in families.

COURSE It occurs in people who are perfectly healthy, and has a marked tendency to recur over the years. It is not infectious, and does not affect the person internally. It will be diagnosed early in the course of the disease, as it is not easily mistaken for other skin complaints. the condition can gradually clear in about three months, but in more severe cases, it may always be present in varying degrees.

EFFECTS Psoriasis is an unsightly skin condition which mainly affects the elbows, knees, scalp, and abdomen. It sometimes affects the fingers, particularly the nails, but never the face. Affected areas are leathery, raised and red, and are covered with rough white scales. Patients can feel very conscious of unsightly areas, and may have to cover themselves with long sleeves, stockings, etc. In extreme cases the condition causes much distress. The disease seems to be linked with emotional upset and conflict.

TREATMENT Application of lotions and ointments to the affected areas, and ultra violet irradiation.

People Likely to be In Touch

In Hospital Dermatologist, social worker for skin unit/clinic.
At Home General practitioner.

Help Needed

Not likely to be the presenting problem on referral to community workers, but may be part of a more complex picture. People will need understanding and help with the distress this disease causes.

Resources

Psoriasis Association,
7 Milton Street,
Northampton NN2 7JG.
Telephone 0604 711129
Promotes research, educates, gives information and social contact for sufferers. Local branches and self help groups.

Pulmonary Tuberculosis

The Medical Condition

AGE OF ONSET Any age.

CAUSE Infection of the lungs by the tubercle bacillus. May be transmitted by direct contact with a sufferer.

COURSE At first the infection is localized to a small area of lung (a spot). The course varies. In most cases the body puts up resistance to the infection, but cavities may form in the lungs and if untreated patients can quickly become very ill. They may cough up blood. Elderly people may have no symptoms for years, except a cough, but may nevertheless be infectious to others. Nowadays most patients respond satisfactorily to treatment and the disease is seldom fatal.

EFFECTS There may be fever, cough, sweating at night, loss of weight, and general weakness. Overcrowding and malnutrition, other illness, and psychological problems increase the patient's distress, and worsen the outlook.

TREATMENT Combinations of drugs are now very effective. There may need to be a period in hospital and months off work. Prevention however, is the factor which has diminished the incidence of the disease. Good housing, improved public and child health, and mass radiography have radically changed the situation. It is a notifiable infectious disease – that is it must be reported to the Community Physician. A routine check by the Health Visitor from the Chest Clinic is then carried out among the family and contacts such as work or school mates. Where necessary treatment or vaccination (BCG) is offered.

People Likely to be In Touch

In Hospital Chest physician, paediatrician, health visitor (Chest Clinic), social worker.

At Home General practitioner, community physician, health visitor from Chest Clinic.

Help Needed

The incidence of pulmonary tuberculosis may be related to a variety of social problems such as poverty, overcrowding, and bad housing. Families may still regard it with fear and feel it as a stigma. There can be particular guilt where, for example, a grandmother may have infected a child. Work should be in close co-operation with hospital clinic, where there will be support for rehousing and advice on all aspects.

CHECK LIST DHSS Benefits. Rehousing. Convalescence/Holiday. Voluntary grants.

Resources

Chest, Heart and Stroke Association,
Tavistock House (North),
Tavistock Square,
London WC1H 9JE.
Telephone 01 387 3012
Promotes research and wider knowledge, educational literature, cassettes.

Raynaud's Disease

The Medical Condition

AGE OF ONSET Usually young adults, mostly women.

CAUSE Unknown. May be a sign of internal disease. Skilled handworkers or musicians and people working with vibrating tools are susceptible. There is often a psychological element involved.

COURSE The blood vessels supplying the hands (and sometimes feet) suffer attacks of spasm, which virtually shut off the blood supply to the fingers for minutes or hours. If the patient does not respond to treatment, these attacks will recur indefinitely.

EFFECTS When exposed to cold the fingers become dead, pale, sometimes with blue mottling. They are painful and clumsy and remain so until the hands are warmed. Then the skin may become red, tingling, and burning.

TREATMENT Sometimes the condition responds to drugs which control the spasm. If this does not work and the attacks are severe and persistent, a surgical operation can be performed on the neck (cervical sympathectomy). This cuts the nerve supply to the affected blood vessels. Patients often have to wear gloves, even indoors, and have to take special precautions against cold conditions.

People Likely to be In Touch

In Hospital General physician, neurosurgeon, social worker.
At Home General practitioner, health visitor.

Help Needed

This condition is principally one where daily tasks and employment may be affected. Patients may need help with changing from outdoor to indoor jobs, or to work where their hands are less involved. Housewives and young mothers might have difficulty in coping and need practical assistance. They are often paricularly sensitive people who are unable to cope with stress. They may be accessible to counselling for social or emotional problems.

CHECK LIST DHSS Benefits. Disablement Resettlement Officer. Home Help. Day Nursery. Playgroup, etc.

Schizophrenia

The Medical Condition

AGE OF ONSET Usually young adults (more men than women).

CAUSE Unknown. There is a hereditary factor.

COURSE Schizophrenia is a term which should not be taken to refer to a single condition but a number of related states, all of which to some degree involve the fragmentation or disordering of the normal personality and/or perceptual experience. Symptoms develop gradually and tend to recur in episodes, lasting for a few weeks or months. Occasionally severe stress can cause a transient schizophrenic episode, but usually the disease is long lasting. However, symptoms do reduce in intensity and the term 'burnt out schizophrenic' is then used.

EFFECTS Disorder of thoughts which result in delusions, hallucinations, and abnormalities of speech. These may be directly linked with behavioural disturbances, e.g. patient may act upon a delusional belief, or in response to orders from hallucinatory voices, or other outside influences. Abnormalities of mood include depression, exaltation, irritability, and anxiety. Patients often feel paranoid and suspicious. In some cases there is a flattening of mood, with a wooden facial expression, dull tone of voice, and lack of gestures. At times there may be aggressive outbursts, but normally the schizophrenic patient becomes a quiet withdrawn person, often undernourished and neglected looking, lacking in energy and motivation, and socially withdrawn.

TREATMENT By tablets (Largactil, Melleril and other phenothiazines, long acting 'depot' injections such as Modicate). These are now very effective in improving symptoms, but their value in controlling the course of the disease is doubtful. Sometimes psychotherapy is used.

People Likely to be In Touch

In Hospital Psychiatric team – doctor, nursing staff, psychologist, occupational therapist, social worker.

At Home General practitioner, community psychiatric nurse, day hospital, occupational therapy out-patients.

It becomes increasingly difficult for patients to maintain normal social relationships or hold down a job. Family and friends find it harder and harder to 'get through' and have to suffer coldness of manner and detachment of interest. Families may feel constantly apprehensive, wondering when a fresh episode will occur, which could lead to abnormal behaviour. All kinds of social problems inevitably dog this illness. There may be family/marital breakdown, unemployment, accommodation difficulties, poverty, child care, and adolescent problems. Help must be in conjunction with the staff of the psychiatric unit and the primary health care team, and all care and support planned and shared. Social workers may be asked to take part in compulsory admission to hospital under the *Mental Health Act 1959*.

CHECK LIST DHSS Benefits. Holidays. Group Homes. Voluntary Hostels. Lodgings. Voluntary help. Social activities.

Resources

National Association for Mental Health (MIND),
22 Harley Street,
London W1N 2ED.
Telephone 01 637 0741
Advisory and casework service for mental illness. Local Relatives Support Groups – affiliated to MIND.

Mental After Care Association,
Eagle House,
110 Jermyn Street,
London SW1Y 6HB.
Telephone 01 839 5953
Provides hostels, long-term care, and recuperative holidays for people after discharge from mental hospital.

National Schizophrenia Fellowship,
78-9 Victoria Road,
Surbiton,
Surrey KT6 4NS.
Telephone 01 390 3651
Society run by and for relatives. Gives advice and help. Local groups.

Richmond Fellowship,
8 Addison Road,
London W14 8DL.
Telephone 01 603 6373
Provides hostel accommodation and therapeutic group living for young people with psychiatric problems.

National Association for Voluntary Hostels,
33 Long Acre,
London WC2E 9LA.
Telephone 01 836 0193
Will help with placement of single homeless people.

Shingles
(Herpes Zoster)

The Medical Condition

AGE OF ONSET Any age, but more commonly in adults.

CAUSE A virus infection related to that of chicken pox.

COURSE The virus affects nerve roots causing very severe stinging pain in the skin served by the particular nerves. The acute phase may be very uncomfortable, and the long-term effect of nerve pain can continue for months or even years.

EFFECTS The patient may feel ill and have a raised temperature in the early stage of the illness. Little chickenpox-like blisters appear on the skin over the areas where the pain is felt. A common site is on the head, over the eye or in a band around the waistline. The condition can endanger the eye and the persistent neuralgic pricking pain can render the patient suicidal. When the blisters are finally healed there may be scarring and persistent pain.

TREATMENT Various anti-viral remedies either painted on the skin or in tablet form may be used. Sometimes special Pain Clinics can help with the residual pain by blocking the affected nerves with a permanent anaesthetic.

People Likely to be In Touch

In Hospital Physician, neurologist, special pain unit, social worker.

At Home General practitioner, health visitor, district nurse, home help, day hospital/centre.

Help Needed

This condition is likely to arise as part of the problems of elderly people. Isolation and loneliness can make pain more difficult to tolerate and sufferers with persistent after effects may need encouragement and support to return to normal activities. Depression is very common during and after shingles and practical help such as home help or voluntary visiting and outings may be of great value.

CHECK LIST Home Help. Volunteer. Day Care. Convalescence/Holiday.

Resources

See General Organizations for the Disabled and Elderly (page 133).

Spastics

(Cerebral Palsy)

The Medical Condition

AGE OF ONSET Birth.

CAUSE Shortage of oxygen during birth, or birth injury.

COURSE Allowing for growth and development, disability remains static through life.

EFFECTS Can be totally dependent, with constant involuntary writhing movements of limbs and speech difficulty. Often wheelchair bound and sometimes mental development is retarded. On the other hand, can be very independent and degrees of the disability vary between these two extremes.

TREATMENT Palliative and educative. Physiotherapy, occupational therapy, and speech therapy can be helpful.

People Likely to be In Touch

In Hospital Paediatrician, social worker, physiotherapist, occupational therapist, paediatric assessment centre.

At Home General practitioner, health visitor, Education Department, Spastics Society, Day Centres, employer.

Help Needed

This condition is not always recognizable at birth and therefore the primary health care team may be the first to be involved. The family faces a long-term problem with a disabled child and help will be needed from health, education, and social services. There is a need for regular assessment and forward planning. The Spastic Society have a social work service.

CHECK LIST DHSS Benefits – Attendance Allowance, Mobility Allowance. Aids and Adaptations – refer to occupational therapist. Short/long term residential care. Day Care. Holidays. Voluntary help.

Resources

Spastics Society,
12 Park Crescent,
London W1N 4EQ.
Telephone 01 636 5020

Provides facilities for assessment, treatment, education, training, sheltered housing, and residential care of spastics in sixty establishments. Wide range of advice services. Holidays. Publishes a monthly magazine *Spastics News* and has own social work service.
See Local Groups.

Star Organization for Spastics,
The Star Centre,
Ullenwood,
Cheltenham,
Gloucestershire.
Provides further education and training for young adults of sixteen plus.

Spina Bifida, Hydrocephalus

The Medical Condition

AGE OF ONSET Birth.

CAUSE Unknown. There is a risk that more than one affected child may be born to a family.

COURSE Spina Bifida is one of the commonest congenital disabilities. The spine fails to develop properly and cystic swelling which involves the spinal cord and nerves is present on the back at birth. Hydrocephalus – 'water on the brain', is also present in 85 per cent of these babies. This is a high pressure of fluid in the brain. The course depends on whether the baby survives beyond the first few weeks, and in cases of hydrocephalus whether surgery is carried out to drain the excess fluid. Nearly all children will be left with a degree of disability, some very severe.

EFFECTS Many spina bifida children have some paralysis from birth, usually of the legs, so that walking is a problem. Limbs can be deformed or without feeling, and there is often very little control of bladder or bowels. Recurrent infections in the urinary tract are common, and the kidneys may fail to function. In addition, those children who have had surgery for hydrocephalus may develop infection or obstruction in the inserted valve ('shunt').

TREATMENT Pre-natal screening, including taking a sample of amniotic fluid (surrounding the foetus) can identify most spina bifida babies before birth. Therefore, fewer live children are likely to be born with this condition. Babies may undergo surgery in the first months of life to prevent hydrocephalus. A valve is inserted to drain the excess fluid from the brain, and this valve may have to be replaced from time to time as the child grows. Incontinence of urine can be dealt with by surgery. The urinary tract is diverted and an ileostomy is performed. (See page 37 for ileostomy.) Genetic counselling may be arranged by the hospital team.

People Likely to be In Touch

In Hospital Paediatrician, neurosurgeon, orthopaedic or general surgeon, physiotherapist, social worker, paediatric assessment centre, stoma sister.

At Home General practitioner, health visitor, district nurse, domiciliary occupational therapist, special schooling – Education department, school counsellor, stoma sister and clinic.

Help Needed

Workers in the community are likely to come across families with a spina bifida child, after the first impact of shock and distress. Work with the family should be in close co-operation with the hospital team, and the general practitioner and health visitor. The baby may die soon after birth and parents need counselling and support through their bereavement. Medical decisions to offer or withhold treatment are very difficult and delicate. Parents will therefore be very closely associated with the hospital staff at these times, but they may need support beyond that which the hospital can provide. Where the child survives, he and his family face all the practical and emotional problems of handicap. Parents will experience continuing anxiety and sometimes face a heavy nursing task. They can feel restricted and depressed and may need 'time off'. Where no immediate family are available baby sitters and self help groups may be useful. Schooling brings fresh problems, and education, social, and health workers must co-operate and make joint plans for the child with the family.

CHECK LIST DHSS Benefits – Attendance Allowance, Mobility Allowance. Parents groups. Education Department. Aids and Adaptations – refer to domiciliary occupational therapist. Holidays. Programmed relief residential care. Voluntary Society.

Resources

Association for Spina Bifida and Hydrocephalus,
Tavistock House (North),
Tavistock Square,
London WC1H 9HJ.
Telephone 01 388 1382
Advice and financial help available. Local branches for support to parents.

Spinal Cord Injuries/ Disease

The Medical Condition

AGE OF ONSET Any age.

CAUSE The spine is made up of thirty bones with the spinal cord running down the centre. These bones are named in four sections from the top – cervical, thoracic, lumbar, and sacral. If the spinal cord is damaged, paralysis (partial or complete) will occur below the point of damage.
Paraplegia – paralysis of legs and lower part of body.
Quadraplegia }
Tetraplegia } Paralysis of all four limbs.

COURSE This is dependent on the cause. It may be a gradual or sudden onset due to disease or paralysis occurring following accident or injury.

EFFECTS After the initial effects of the illness or accident, the patient is usually confined to wheelchair living. The majority are not ill, but may have a sensory loss of pain, heat, and cold in the affected limbs. There will be problems of incontinence and sometimes spasticity. Some have breathing difficulties and are prone to chest and urinary infections. Pressure sores are a permanent hazard. Some, mainly younger patients, lead an extremely active life, despite immense physical and psychological difficulties.

TREATMENT At first patients need constant care and prevention of complications. Physiotherapy and occupational therapy, within the limits of the general condition, will help to promote general health and independence.

People Likely to be In Touch

In Hospital Spinal Injuries Unit (Regional) for first assessment and treatment plan, neurologist, orthopaedic surgeon, physiotherapist, occupational therapist, social worker.

At Home General practitioner, district nurse, health visitor, domiciliary occupational therapist, day hospital/centre, Disablement Resettlement Officer.

Help Needed

Most patients will be referred when they are returning to the community from a special unit or rehabilitation centre. This can be a very difficult and sometimes depressing time for both patient and family. They will need practical help and emotional support, and many need time before they are willing to participate in life as disabled people. Children of disabled parents may need help in their own right. The family should have access to an agreed key worker, so that they know to whom to turn in problems or crises. Sexual counselling may be helpful.

CHECK LIST DHSS Benefits – Attendance Allowance, Mobility Allowance, Motability, Non-contributory Housewives Allowance. Housing. Aids and Adaptations – refer to occupational therapist. Education. Employment – Disabled Resettlement Officer. Home Help. Meals on Wheels. Day Care. Temporary or permanent residential care. Holidays. Domiciliary Care Attendant. Voluntary help.

Resources

Spinal Injuries Association,
5 Crowndale Road,
London NW1.
Telephone 01 388 6840
Publish a newsletter and a series of helpful pamphlets for professionals and families which cover all aspects of treatment and rehabilitation.

General Organizations for the Disabled (see page 133).

Still's Disease

The Medical Condition

AGE OF ONSET Childhood – as early as two years of age.

CAUSE Unknown. It is related to adult rheumatoid arthritis and can imitate it exactly.

COURSE The illness begins slowly and is progressively disabling. It is characterized by attacks and remissions until the picture of established rheumatoid arthritis emerges.

EFFECTS The child suffers a series of feverish illnesses which leave him debilitated. The small joints (fingers, hands, wrists) are painful and swollen and as time goes on these swellings do not disappear after attacks. Some wasting or deformity may develop.

TREATMENT This is the same as for rheumatoid arthritis. Cortisone type drugs are often used. These may have side effects and stunt the child's growth, or delay his sexual development. Physiotherapy may help to prevent immobility and sometimes surgery is used to straighten contracted limbs. Pain killing drugs are needed throughout.

People Likely to be In Touch

In Hospital Rheumatologist, paediatrician, orthopaedic surgeon, physiotherapist, occupational therapist, hospital teacher, social worker.

At Home General practitioner, health visitor, district nurse, domiciliary occupational therapist, education department, careers department (special adviser for disabled school leavers).

Help Needed

These children face the life long problems of disabling disease with the consequent effects on the lives of the parents and other siblings. Admission to hospital isolates the child from his normal environment and affects his education and the achievement of normal milestones. It is important to liaise with the hospital team, primary health care team, and school/education department. There is a need for continuous assessment and forward planning for each stage with the parents, child, and other workers involved. The child himself may need special counselling, particularly during adolescence.

CHECK LIST DHSS Benefits – Attendance Allowance, Mobility Allowance. Aids and Adaptations – refer to domiciliary occupational therapist. Education Department – special schooling. Holidays for child/parents/siblings.

Resources

As for Rheumatoid Arthritis.
Helpful Organizations for Children (see page 136).

Stroke

(Cerebrovascular Accident)

The Medical Condition

AGE OF ONSET Middle to old age, but can happen earlier.

CAUSE Damage to the brain due to a bleed, a clot, or a blockage of an artery. Associated with narrowing of the arteries and high blood pressure.

COURSE The onset is usually sudden and often devastating. There may be loss of consciousness and heavy breathing. The first week is the critical period. Patients may have some paralysis of the arm or leg on one side and this is known as hemiplegia. There is always a risk of a further stroke. Many people make a good recovery.

EFFECTS *Immediate* Unconscious, breathing difficulty, loss of speech, affected sight, incontinence, confusion. In need of medical help and total nursing care.

Long term The patient may be left with paralysis and speech difficulties. Patients are usually unaware of paralysed side and feel it does not belong to them. Some suffer a personality change or go through a period of depression. Incontinence may be a problem.

TREATMENT Expert nursing, physiotherapy, occupational therapy, and speech therapy to achieve maximum rehabilitation. Many patients go to special rehabilitation units or stroke units, where a team approach is of vital importance to the resettlement of the patient, concentrating on the family abilities as much as those of the patient.

People Likely to be In Touch

In Hospital Physician, geriatrician, neurologist, specialist in rehabilitation, psychologist, physiotherapist, occupational therapist, social worker.

At Home General practitioner, district nurse, health visitor, stroke club, day hospital/centre, domiciliary occupational therapist.

Help Needed

Referral may come from hospital for help in resettling patient at home. On first returning home the effects of the disability become much more apparent, as does the impact on the family, and a period of frustration and depression is almost inevitable. The breadwinner may not be able to return to work or the housewife to her former role. They will need practical help and emotional support. Loss of speech or difficulty in communicating are particularly distressing and frustrating.

CHECK LIST DHSS Benefits – Attendance Allowance, Mobility, Motability, Invalid Care Allowance, Non-Contributory Housewives Allowance. Day Care/Hospital. Housing. Aids and Adaptations – refer to occupational therapist. Employment – refer to Disablement Resettlement Officer. Home Help. Meals on Wheels. Periodic/permanent residential care. Holidays. Voluntary help.

Resources

Chest, Heart and Stroke Association,
Tavistock House (North),
Tavistock Square,
London WC1H 9J1.
Telephone 01 387 3012
Promotes research and wider knowledge, educational literature, cassettes.

Some local groups and health/social service personnel run 'Stroke Clubs'.

Syringomyelia

The Medical Condition

AGE OF ONSET Early adult life; males predominate.

CAUSE Unknown.

COURSE The illness begins insidiously and progresses slowly. Some patients are able to lead a relatively normal life. However, after middle age they are liable to become worse and because of their vulnerability to infection are not likely to reach old age.

EFFECTS Patients first notice that their hands are becoming thinner, and they are burning or cutting their fingers without noticing the heat or pain (although light touch can still be felt). Sometimes a blister or sore is the first sign that anything has happened. The loss of feeling may extend to other parts of the body including the tongue. In the later stages the legs may become stiff and weak.

TREATMENT None. A very minute proportion of cases can be helped by surgery.

People Likely to be In Touch

In Hospital Neurologist, general physician, social worker, occupational therapist.

At Home General practitioner, domiciliary occupational therapist, district nurse.

Help Needed

Check with hospital social worker. Help may not be necessary in the community unless symptoms become severe, with consequent family and emotional problems. Particularly where patients are living alone, special help may be needed to guard against the risk of burns and cuts, i.e. water temperatures, sharp edges, cookers etc. The domiciliary occupational therapist should be asked to help.

CHECK LIST DHSS Benefits – Invalid Care Allowance, Attendance Allowance, Mobility Allowance, Disabled Housewives Allowance. Home Help. Meals on Wheels. Day Care. Short term residential care. Holiday.

Resources

There are no resources specifically linked with this condition. See General Organizations for the Disabled (page 133).

Trigeminal Neuralgia

(Tic Douloureux)

The Medical Condition

AGE OF ONSET More common in older people.

CAUSE Unknown. The trigeminal nerve, which is the sensory nerve to the face, develops a tendency to transmit false signals to the brain which are felt as attacks of the most severe lancinating pain.

COURSE There are clusters of attacks of one-sided facial pain which can be very distressing. Unless treated, attacks occur more and more frequently with fewer periods of remission.

EFFECTS Attacks are sometimes brought on by the normal movements of the face, i.e. talking and eating, or by exposure to cold wind or damp conditions. People can live in terror of the next bout of pain.

TREATMENT Usually the attacks can be prevented by regular medication. Prompt treatment is essential. In more severe cases the nerve can be injected or severed, leaving one side of the face without feeling.

People Likely to be In Touch

In Hospital Neurologist, neurosurgeon, social worker, special pain clinic.

At Home General practitioner, health visitor.

Help Needed

This condition may show as part of a more complex elderly problem. The effects of the acute pain should not be underestimated. Elderly people can be totally incapacitated during attacks and may need short term relief and help. It is essential to ensure medical attention and routine medication.

CHECK LIST DHSS Benefits. Volunteers. Home Help. Meals on Wheels. Day Care/Hospital. Periodic residential care.

Resources

See General Organizations for the Elderly (page 133).

Ulcerative Colitis

The Medical Condition

AGE OF ONSET Mostly before the age of thirty.

CAUSE A recurrent inflammation of the bowel, probably due to an unusual reaction to the bacteria that are always present. It is also associated with certain types of personality, i.e. over conscientious, obsessional, immature.

COURSE The disease usually starts insidiously and can remain hardly noticeable. It may become so acute as to threaten the life of the patient. Mild cases can completely recover. More severe cases after radical treatment can live a healthy life but relapse is always a possibility.

EFFECTS Attacks of abdominal pain and diarrhoea of varying severity, passing blood, mucus, and pus. The constant diarrhoea leads to weakness, loss of weight, and anaemia. The disease can sometimes be complicated by chronic rheumatic conditions.

TREATMENT An important factor in treatment is an understanding of the patient's personality and problems. Hospital admission may be necessary and it can help the patient to be out of the home environment. Treatment varies according to the severity of the disease. Drugs and blood transfusions are given. In some cases surgery may be necessary, leading to colostomy. Attention needs to be paid to diet.

People Likely to be In Touch

In Hospital Physician, gastro-enterologist, surgeon, social worker, dietician, occupational therapist, psychiatrist/ psychologist.

At Home General practitioner, district nurse, Disablement Resettlement Officer.

Help Needed

Because of the recognized emotional content of the disease, there are likely to be personal or family problems. There will often be loss of employment and curtailment of social life. Link with hospital or primary health care team. Long term supportive casework may be needed.

CHECK LIST DHSS Benefits – diet allowance, Home Help, holidays for patients and family, convalescence.

Resources

See Colostomy and Ileostomy – page 37.

Veneral Disease I
Gonorrhoea

The Medical Condition

AGE OF ONSET From the age of puberty. Babies at birth.

CAUSE Infection of the genitals by a micro-organism called the gonococcus. Almost always transmitted through sexual intercourse with an infected person. Babies can become infected by their mothers during labour.
NB. 'NSU' or non-specific urethritis is an almost equally common venereal disease with the same signs, but the gonococcus is not found in the discharge. It may be due to a virus, and it can produce a form of generalized arthritis which can last many months. (Reiter's Syndrome.)

COURSE AND EFFECTS Symptoms appear up to ten days following infection. There is pain on passing urine, and a discharge. Symptoms may be so mild that the disease can go unnoticed. If the infection is untreated it may spread, and have serious results, such as permanent infertility in women, and inflammation of the prostate gland in men.

TREATMENT By injection of antibiotics, usually penicillin, which is effective in a matter of hours. Patients are then tested over a period of time for freedom from infection. Clinics or Centres are easily accessible to patients and some are held after working hours. Confidentiality is carefully guarded because of the nature of the disease and its social implications. One of the most important aspects of treatment is that of finding the patient's sexual partner, who may have passed on the infection, or contracted it. This may be extremely difficult if the relationship has been a casual one, or if there are complicated marital or social problems. Attached to most clinics are special workers 'contact tracers' who encourage contacts to attend clinic for testing.

People Likely to be In Touch

Once the patient is in touch with the clinic or centre, the whole matter is usually handled by the venereologist and clinic team.

Help Needed

There is an alarming increase in the incidence of venereal disease, especially among teenagers. It is a social problem and still holds implications of morality and guilt. Promiscuity can be seen as part of an adolescent rebellion. Children in trouble are particularly vulnerable and may be reluctant to seek help. It is important to ensure that young people are properly informed and know where to go for treatment.

Resources

Special clinic in the District General Hospital. Information about local treatment centres available from the Community Health Sector of the Area or District Health Authority.

Venereal Disease II Syphilis

The Medical Condition

AGE OF ONSET From the age of puberty. Can be congenital (passed from mother to unborn child).

CAUSE An infection of the genitals by a micro-organism called the spirochaete. Almost always contracted through sexual intercourse with an infected person.
NB. Syphilis is a potentially more dangerous disease than gonorrhoea, though it is now a much more rare condition.

COURSE AND EFFECTS The incubation period is one to six weeks. The first stage is characterized by the appearance on the penis or the labia of a hard, painless red spot, which enlarges to form an ulcer. Because of the lack of pain at this stage, the disease can go unnoticed and the ulcer heals spontaneously. Diagnosis can be confirmed by a blood test called the Wasserman test. The second stage, in six to twelve weeks' time, is characterized by mild feverishness, lassitude, headache, and a non-itching rash. Again the diagnosis can be confirmed by blood test, but the condition can be missed and the symptoms subside without treatment. If untreated or inadequately treated, the third stage may appear five to twenty years later. It may show in various forms of illness affecting the nervous system, blood vessels, and bladder. The outlook is serious. There can be a gradual deterioration in personality, emotional control, and concentration, leading to complete dementia and paralysis. This is known as General Paralysis of the Insane (GPI).

TREATMENT The infection is curable in the first and second stages by penicillin and other antibiotics. Because of the improvement in diagnosis and efficient treatment, the third stage is rarely seen. The same methods of 'contact tracing' apply – see Venereal Disease I (page 128).

People Likely to be In Touch

Once the patient is in touch with the clinic or centre, the whole matter is usually handled by the venereologist and clinic team.

Help Needed

There is an alarming increase in the incidence of venereal disease, especially among teenagers. It is a social problem and still holds implications of morality and guilt. Promiscuity can be seen as part of an adolescent rebellion. Children in trouble are particularly vulnerable and may be reluctant to seek help. It is important to ensure that young people are properly informed, and know where to go for treatment.

Resources

Special clinic in the District General Hospital. Information about local treatment centres available from the Community Health Sector of the Area or District Health Authority.

Further Reading

The Handicapped Person in the Community David M. Boswell and Janet M. Wingrove (London: Tavistock Publications, 1974)

Take Care of Your Elderly Relative J. A. Muir Gray and Heather McKenzie (London: Allen & Unwin, 1980)

Our Elders J. A. Muir Gray and Gordon Wilcock (Oxford: Oxford University Press, 1981)

Care of the Elderly Mentally Infirm Bernard Isaacs and Barbara Gray (London: Tavistock Publications, 1979)

The Sexual Side of Handicap W. F. R. Stewart (Cambridge: Woodhead-Faulkner, 1979)

Entitled to Love W. Greengross (London: National Marriage Guidance Council, 1976)

Holes in the Welfare Net Maureen Oswin (London: Bedford Square Press, 1978)

A Life Apart E. J. Miller and G. V. Gwynne (London: Tavistock Publications, 1974)

The Meaning of Disability Mildred Blaxter (London: Heinemann Educational, 1976)

ABC Services and Information for Disabled People (London: Disablement Income Group, 1977)

Directory for the Disabled Ann Darnbrough and Derek Kinrade (Cambridge: Woodhead-Faulkner, 1979)

Charities Digest Produced by Family Welfare Association (London: Butterworths, 1979)

The following titles appear in a series published by the Oxford University Press:

Asthma – The Facts D. Lane and Anthony Storr

Sexually Transmitted Diseases – The Facts David Barlow

Arthritis and Rheumatism – The Facts J. T. Scott

Cancer – The Facts Sir Ronald Bodley Scott

Migraine – The Facts F. Clifford Rose and M. Gawel

Multiple Sclerosis – The Facts Brian Matthews

Coronary Heart Disease – The Facts J. P. Shillingford

Kidney Disease – The Facts Stewart Cameron

Epilepsy – The Facts Anthony Hopkins

Stroke – The Facts F. Clifford Rose and R. Capildeo

Alcoholism – The Facts D. W. Goodwin

Breast Cancer – The Facts Michael Baum

General Organizations for the Disabled and Elderly

Age Concern England (National Old People's Welfare Council),
Bernard Sunley House,
60 Pitcairn Road,
Mitcham,
Surrey CR4 3LL
Telephone 01 640 5431

Promotes welfare for old people. Local Committees. Elderly Invalids Fund and Old People's Advisory Service. Gives financial help and advice to elderly people.

British Red Cross Society,
9 Grosvenor Crescent,
London SW1X 7EJ
Telephone 01 235 5454

Community welfare services for the disabled. Local branches.

Community Service Volunteers,
237 Pentonville Road,
London N1 9NJ
Telephone 01 278 6601

Provides volunteer help for holidays or relief care.

Disability Alliance,
5 Netherhall Gardens,
London NW3
Telephone 01 794 1536

Works to achieve a comprehensive income scheme. Local groups

Disabled Living Foundation,
346 Kensington High Street,
London W14 8NS
Telephone 01 602 2491

Promotes a general information service for the disabled, including aids.

Disabled Drivers' Association,
Ashwellthorpe Hall,
Ashwellthorpe,
Norwich NR16 1EX
Telephone Fundenhall 449

Helps disabled people with car conversions, insurance, and all motoring matters.

Disabled Drivers' Motor Club Ltd.,
9 Park Parade,
Gunnersbury Avenue,
London W3 9BD
Telephone 01 993 6454

Offers facilities and advice on all aspects of motoring. Reduced RAC subscription.

Disablement Income Group,
Attlee House,
Toynbee Hall,
28 Commercial Street,
London E1 6LR
Telephone 01 247 2128

Pressure group campaigning to improve the economic and social position of disabled people. Local groups.

Invalids at Home Trust,
23 Farm Avenue,
London NW2
Telephone 01 452 2074

Provides financial help for disabled at home.

Leonard Cheshire Foundation,
7 Market Mews,
London W1Y 8HP
Telephone 01 499 2665

Provides residential accommodation for disabled people.

National Council for the Single Woman and her Dependants,
29 Chilworth Mews,
London W2 3RG
Telephone 01 262 1451

Assists single women caring for elderly relatives. Local branches.

PHAB (Physically Handicapped and Able Bodied),
42 Devonshire Street,
London W1N 1LN
Telephone 01 637 7475

Integrated activities for physically handicapped and able bodied people. Local groups.

Soldiers, Sailors and Airmens Families Association (SSAFA),
27 Queen Anne's Gate,
London SW1H 9BZ
Telephone 01 839 4131

Advice and welfare services for families of service and ex-service men and women. Local branches.

SPOD Committee on Sexual and Personal Relationships of the Disabled,
Brook House,
2-16 Torrington Place,
London WC1E 7HN
Telephone 01 637 4712

Promotes awareness of the problems and factual information and advice to handicapped people and others concerned. Enquiries by letter to SPOD.

Many of the Organizations mentioned in this book have Scottish headquarters or branches.
Information on these available from:
Scottish Information Service for the Disabled,
18 Claremont Crescent,
Edinburgh EH7 4QD
Telephone 031 556 3882

Helpful Organizations for Handicapped or Invalid Children

Association of Parents of Vaccine Damaged Children,
2 Church Street,
Shipston-on-Stour,
Warwickshire CV36 4AP
Telephone Shipston-on-Stour 61595

Represents and campaigns for these children.

Child Poverty Action Group,
1 Macklin Street,
London WC2B 5NH
Telephone 01 242 3225

Promotes relief of poverty and advises on welfare benefit problems.

Down's Children's Association,
Quinborne Community Centre,
Ridgacre Road,
Quinton,
Birmingham B32 2TW
Telephone 021 427 1374

Advice with developmental management of mongol children and the promotion of research into care and education.

Handicapped Children's Aid Committee,
154 Anson Road,
London NW2
Telephone 01 452 2627

Help given in a wide variety of ways.

Invalid Children's Aid Association,
126 Buckingham Palace Road,
London SW1W 9SB
Telephone 01 730 9891

Free help and advice for parents with handicapped children.

Lady Hoare Trust for Physically Disabled Children,
7 North Street,
Midhurst,
West Sussex GU29 9DJ
Telephone 073 081 3696

Welfare support of every kind to families. Holiday homes.

Malcolm Sargent Cancer Fund For Children,
56 Redcliffe Square,
London SW10 9HQ
Telephone 01 373 5861.

Gives financial help.

National Association for the Welfare of Children in Hospital,
7 Exton Street,
London SE1 8VE
Telephone 01 261 1738

General help to children in hospital, and their parents.

National Children's Home,
Principal – The Rev. Gordon E. Barritt,
85 Highbury Park,
London N5 1UD
Telephone 01 226 2033

Two residential schools for physically handicapped children at Harpenden, Herts, and at Chipping Norton, Oxon. Two homes for severely subnormal children, and three schools for ESN children.

National Society for Brain Damaged Children,
Hon. Secretary, 35 Larchmore Drive,
Hall Green,
Birmingham 28
Telephone 021 777 4284

Assessment facilities and information.

National Society for Mentally Handicapped Children and Adults (MENCAP),
117-123 Golden Lane,
London EC1Y 0RT
Telephone 01 253 9433

Local branches. Regional offices. Gateway Clubs for Seniors and Juniors. Residential homes. Welfare visitors.

Shaftesbury Society,
Shaftesbury House,
112 Regency Street,
London SW1P 4AX
Telephone 01 834 2656

Five residential schools for physically disabled children, four homes for physically handicapped young men. Some club and holiday centres.

The Family Fund,
Joseph Rowntree Memorial Trust,
PO Box 50,
York YO3 6RB

The fund gives assistance to under sixteen-year-old severely handicapped children, with special transport, unusual adaptations and aids, holidays and laundry equipment.

Toy Libraries Association for Handicapped Children,
Seabrook House,
Wyllyotts Manor,
Darkes Lane,
Potters Bar EN6 2HL
Telephone Potters Bar 44571

Seventy libraries lending toys to handicapped children.

See Annual Charities and Director of Grant Making Trusts.
Published by:
Charities Aid Foundation,
48 Pembury Road,
Tonbridge,
Kent TN9 2JD

Who's Who in the Health Service

DOCTORS Although he is entitled to call himself 'doctor' as soon as he has graduated, a doctor still has to spend a year working under supervision in hospital as a house officer or 'houseman' before he can register with the General Medical Council. After registration most doctors either train to become general practitioners or specialize in hospital work.

GENERAL PRACTITIONERS To become a general practitioner the doctor has to undergo a three-year vocational training period which includes one year in a training practice, during which the trainee will have full clinical responsibility for the patients whom he treats. The remainder of the training period is spent in those hospital specialities which are particularly relevant to general practice. After completing training and passing the membership examination of the Royal College of General Practitioners (MRCGP) the doctor may enter general practice. The general practitioner is not an employee of the health authority. He is what is known as an 'independent contractor' and is now under the management of a community physician or 'the principal', that is the senior doctor in the practice.

HOSPITAL DOCTORS The training of hospital doctors takes anything between ten and twelve years from registration to a consultant status. The hospital doctor climbs a ladder, spending about four years on each rung.

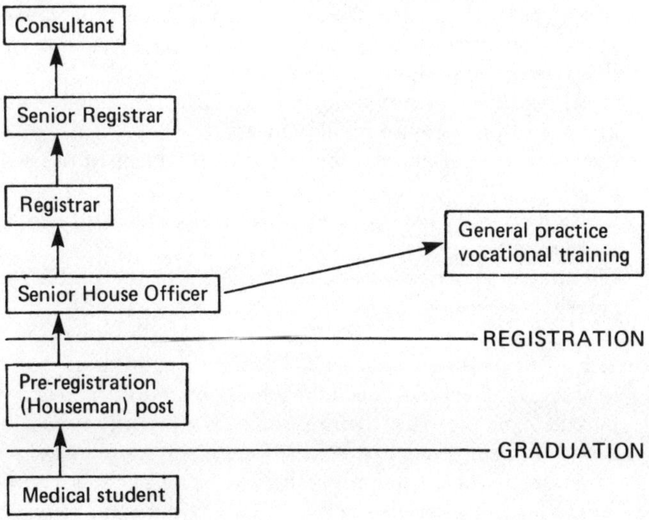

During this training the doctor has to sit two further examinations for his higher professional qualification of which the most common are the MRCP (Member of the Royal College of Physicians) and FRCS (Fellow of the Royal College of Surgeons). These are usually passed while the doctor is a registrar and as the FRCS entitles a doctor to adopt, or revert to, the title 'Mister' there are many surgeons who are called 'Mister' who are not consultants.

At senior registrar level the hospital doctor specializes and the following are the more common specialities:

SURGICAL SPECIALITIES (SURGEONS) *General surgeons* deal with stomach and bowel problems, breast disorders, hernias, and other less common problems.

Orthopaedic surgeons deal with disorders of bones and joints resulting from accidents and from chronic diseases such as arthritis.

Neurosurgeons operate on the brain and spinal cord.

Vascular surgeons specializes in diseases of the blood vessels. They often also perform renal transplantation.

Cardiac surgeons operate on the heart.

Urologists specialize in kidney and bladder disease.

Obstetricians specialize in pregnancy and childbirth.

Gynaecologists specialize in the diseases of women.

MEDICAL SPECIALITIES (PHYSICIANS) *General Physicians* are trained to diagnose and give medical treatment to the full range of diseases, but usually have a special interest in one or more types of disease.

Rheumatologists deal with the medical aspects of bone and joint disorders.

Neurologists are concerned with the medical aspects of brain and spinal cord disorders such as multiple sclerosis, and with diseases of the peripheral nerves.

Renal physicians or nephrologists, specialize in kidney failure and are responsible for renal dialysis.

Cardiologists specialize in the medical treatment of heart disease.

Consultants in genito-urinary medicine specialize in sexually transmitted diseases.

Consultants in geriatric medicine specialize in the problems of elderly people.

COMMUNITY PHYSICIAN The Community Physician's task is to assess the health needs of the whole community and to try to persuade people to use their resources as efficiently as possible. Some are principally involved in health service management, some are involved in preventive medicine such as running family planning services or by working with health educators, and others are concerned with the needs of client groups which involve many aspects of health and social services, for example elderly people.

NURSES Nursing auxiliaries receive only basic in-service training and are similar to care assistants. There are two types of trained nurse – the State Enrolled Nurse (SEN) and the more highly qualified State Registered Nurse (SRN).

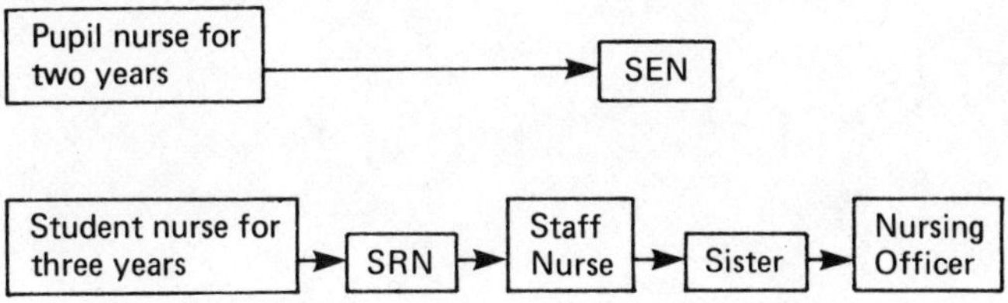

This pattern is the same for both 'general' and psychiatric nurses. Community nurses are of three types – community midwives, district nurses, and health visitors. District nurses are all qualified nurses who receive special training for work in the community. Most of their work is with old people and they concentrate on the more skilled tasks such as giving of insulin injections and the treatment of leg ulcers or bed sores, delegating the general care such as bathing to nursing auxiliaries. Health visitors have a full year of polytechnic education covering social administration, preventive medicine, and human growth and development. Most of their work is with families with young children, but an increasing proportion of their work is with disabled and elderly people. Health visitors and district nurses are members of primary care teams with general practitioners, but they are not accountable to doctors. Each community nurse also works as a member of a community nursing team, accountable to a nursing officer. A consequence of this is that a social worker can approach a health visitor or district nurse directly, without a general practitioner's consent.

OCCUPATIONAL AND PHYSIOTHERAPISTS Diseases have primary and secondary effects. The primary effects are treated by the doctor. The secondary effects result from the immobility which the disease produces, and may be joint stiffness, muscle weakness, and loss of confidence. It is the physiotherapist's task to treat the secondary effects by such methods as exercise, heat, massage etc. Physiotherapists have equipment at their disposal but concentrate on consolidating and developing the patient's residual strength and abilities. The job of the occupational therapist is to teach the patient how to overcome his disability in coping with his environment. For example, she will show the stroke patient easier ways of toiletting, washing, dressing, and the simpler tasks of housekeeping. She will assess and provide aids where necessary, or arrange for structural adaptations to the patient's home.